A Colour Atlas of

Surgical Pathology

W. Guthrie
MBChB, FRCPath

Senior Lecturer in Histopathology
Honorary Consultant Pathologist
Ninewells Hospital and Medical School
University of Dundee

R. Fawkes
FIMLS

Senior Chief Medical Laboratory
Scientific Officer
Department of Pathology
Ninewells Hospital and Medical School
University of Dundee

Wolfe Medical Publications Ltd

Copyright © W. Guthrie, R. Fawkes, 1982
Published by Wolfe Medical Publications Ltd, 1982
Printed by Royal Smeets Offset b.v.,
Weert, Netherlands
ISBN 0 7234 0759 2

This book is one of the titles in the series of
Wolfe Medical Atlases, a series which brings
together probably the world's largest systematic
published collection of diagnostic colour
photographs.
For a full list of Atlases in the series, plus
forthcoming titles and details of our surgical,
dental and veterinary Atlases, please write to
Wolfe Medical Publications Ltd, Wolfe House,
3 Conway Street, London W1P 6HE.

General Editor, Wolfe Medical Atlases:
William F. Walker, FRCS (Edin. and London).

Contents

Preface

This Atlas of surgical pathology contains colour photographs of pathological specimens from patients suffering from conditions presently dealt with by surgeons. Photomicrographs from selected cases are included to give an overall histopathological coverage, sufficient to satisfy the needs of undergraduate and postgraduate students preparing for examinations in pathology, as well as providing the practising histopathologist and surgeon with a ready reference to illustrations of a wide range of common diseases, as well as some of the more uncommon but well-known disorders.

The Atlas is divided into ten chapters each comprising a group of topographical topics (T) corresponding in general to the SNOP classification, devised by the College of American Pathologists.

In each chapter alterations in the various organs are dealt with under eight major SNOP morphological (M) headings – traumatic, congenital, mechanical, inflammatory, degenerative, fine cytological, growth disorder and neoplastic. Where an aetiological agent only is illustrated, the SNOP aetiological (E) number is given.

We have tried to tailor cover according to the importance or frequency of any topic or alteration, and where diagnostic difficulties are well recognised extra space has been allotted. Age, sex, occupation, race and nationality are included in many of the case histories, because they often provide important clues to the correct diagnosis. Included are several examples of tropical diseases from patients who have undergone surgical biopsies. Special techniques such as electronmicroscopy, immunofluorescent microscopy, histochemistry and immunoperoxidase staining are included mainly where they are considered essential for diagnosis. The magnifications quoted for each photomicrograph is that of the original 35 mm transparency. Electronmicrograph magnifications are as stated.

This Atlas is primarily intended to illustrate gross surgical specimens. Therefore, we have restricted the histological coverage of needle and endoscopic biopsies to those relating to actual resected specimens. A few necropsy specimens are included where they appear to be particularly relevant.

The appendix has been compiled as a guide for trainee surgeons and pathologists in the sincere hope that mistakes can be avoided and good relations maintained between theatre and laboratory staff.

Acknowledgements

We thank the following who have helped us to complete this Atlas:
Professor J. Swanson Beck for access to the material in the department
of Pathology in Ninewells Hospital, Dundee, and for his continued
encouragement and interest.

Emeritus Professor A. C. Lendrum, Professor W. W. Park, Dr.
George H. Smith, Mr J. W. Corkhill, Mr D. S. Fraser, Mr W. Slidders
and the late Mr S. M. Morrison through whose continued efforts
valuable material and methods were available to us from Dundee Royal
Infirmary, Maryfield Hospital and Queens College, Dundee. Our
surgical colleagues and operating-theatre staff whose co-operation has
enabled us to prepare the specimens for macroscopic and microscopic
presentation. Our medical colleagues in the Department of Pathology,
Ninewells Hospital, Dundee for their co-operation and for providing
material from cases dealt with by them. The scientific staff of the
Department of Pathology, Ninewells Hospital, Dundee for help in the
preparation of some of the specimens and sections but particularly Mrs
Sheila Gibbs, Mrs Wilma Stewart, Mr George Coghill, Mr Gordon
Milne, Mr Stewart McPherson, Mr Andrew Grant, Mr Alan Webster,
and Mr W. Milne. The secretarial and clerical staff of the Department of
Pathology, Ninewells Hospital, Dundee, especially Miss Jennifer Towns
and Miss Joan Hay. The help of Mrs Eileen Mackenzie who typed the
manuscript is gratefully acknowledged.

1 Integumentary haematological lymphatological systems

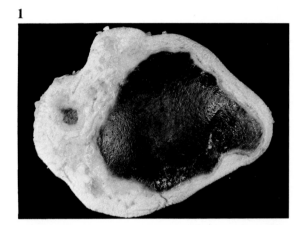

Skin and subcutaneous tissues (T01 – T03)

1 Caustic soda burn (1100) (6 × 6 cm) of forearm from a 44-year-old woman. The specimen was resected to allow grafting.

2 Caustic soda burn (1100) Same case as **1** sliced to show full thickness destruction of dermis and of a 1.5 cm depth of subcutis.

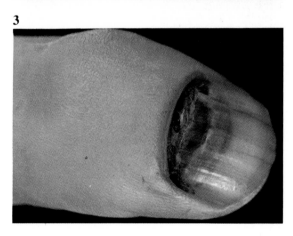

3 Brown discolouration of fingernail (1200) from a 17-year-old youth: it was regarded clinically as malignant melanoma; the finger was amputated. The overall yellow colour is the result of iodine-containing antiseptic used for skin preparation. Histological sections failed to show any neoplasm. The discolouration proved to be partly caused by an alteration in the nail keratin and partly by organising haematoma thought to be related to traumatic disorganisation of the distal interphalangeal joint sustained some months earlier.

4

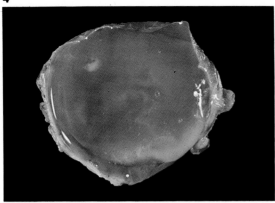

4 Branchial cleft cyst (2534) from the left side of neck, deep to sternomastoid muscle close to the internal jugular vein of a 40-year-old man. The (4×2.2cm) almost translucent cystic mass was received intact and a sample of glistening contents was examined for crystals (see **5**). There was chronic inflammation of the wall in which lymphoid tissue was closely applied to thinned stratified squamous epithelial lining.

5

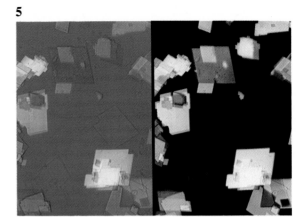

5 Cholesterol crystals from branchial cleft cyst (2534) (shown in **4**) viewed with polarising microscope with (on the left) first order red compensator. The crystals are in plate form often showing the characteristic notch out of one corner. *(×83)*

6

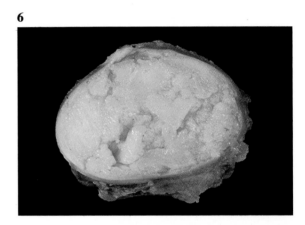

6 Sebaceous cyst from scalp (pilar cyst) (3543) The cyst is 2cm in diameter: the contents are homogeneous and commonly calcify; 90 per cent occur on scalp.

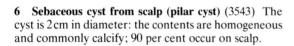

7

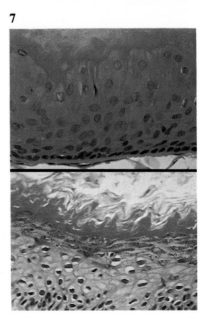

7 Sebaceous cyst and epidermal cyst (3541 + 3543) Sections to show differences in lining. Sebaceous cyst (top) shows epithelial cells without cell bridges, peripheral palisades and innermost cells do not show keratin granules: the keratin formed is hair keratin. Epidermal cyst (bottom) is lined by keratinising stratified squamous epithelium resembling epidermis and its contents of keratin flakes seldom if ever calcify. *(H&E×133)*

8

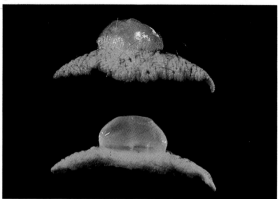

8 Bullous pemphigoid (4080) One of many vesicles developing over nine days on the arms and legs of a 63-year-old labourer. It is subepidermal vesicle 1mm in diameter. Diagnosis was confirmed by demonstrating immunoglobulins on the basement membrane, using immunofluorescent technique.

9

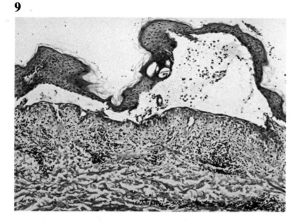

9 Pemphigus vulgaris (4942) Section shows intra-epidermal vesicle with acantholysis. Diagnosis was confirmed by demonstrating immunoglobulins on epidermal cell surface, using immunofluorescent technique. *(H&E × 33)*

10

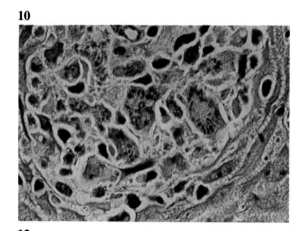

10 Leishmaniasis (tropical sore) (4400) Section shows numerous phagocytes containing the parasites. Imprints or smears made from the ulcer edge give clearer definition of the organism in which a kinetoplast can be made out. *(H&E × 330)*

11

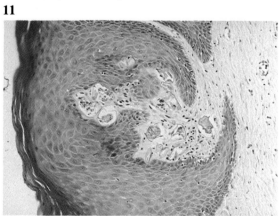

11 Schistosomiasis (4400) The section of a snippet of skin taken to establish the diagnosis in a patient from Zimbabwe, shows eggs with terminal spine (S. haematobium) lying beneath the epidermis and in chronically inflamed fibrosed dermis. *(H&E × 53)*

12

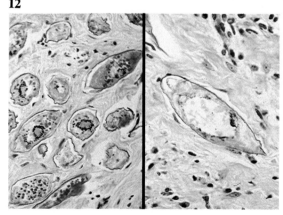

12 Schistosomiasis (4400) Sections showing eggs in cross and longitudinal section: there are plasma cells in the fibrous tissue in these fields; elsewhere there were granulomatous foci, some containing eosinophil polymorphonuclear leucocytes. *(H&E × 83 × 133)*

13

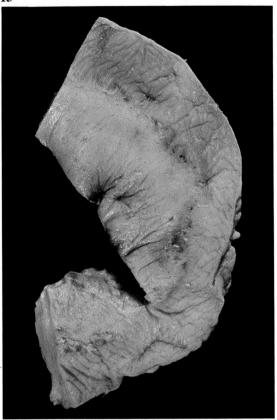

14

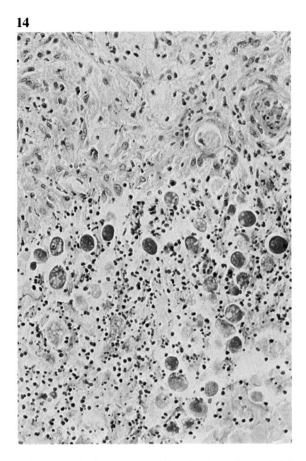

13 Amoebiasis cutis (4410) Part of a wreath of skin excised from the anterior abdominal wall of a merchant seaman whose appendicectomy wound broke down and was followed by progressive destruction of much of the skin of the anterior abdominal wall. The edge of the ulcer was undermined. Ordinary cultures produced a mixed flora and were diagnosed as Meleney's synergistic gangrene. The patient died before the correct diagnosis was established.

14 Amoebiasis cutis (4410) Section shows PAS positive Entamoeba histolytica among exudate under the overhanging subcutaneous tissue which shows non-specific inflammation. *(PAS. H. tartrazine × 83)*

15

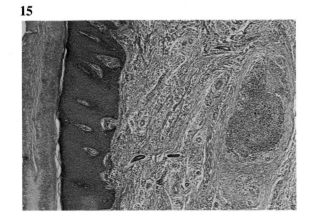

15 Sea urchin granuloma (4410) A nodular painful lesion dating from an injury several months earlier when the young woman trod on a sea urchin on the Mediterranean coast. Section shows deep-seated lesion with suppurative and granulomatous areas containing giant cells of Langhans' type. No microorganisms were identified. Complete excision was curative. *(H&E × 13)*

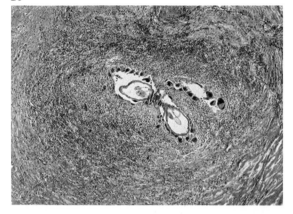

16   Onchocercoma (4410) Section of skin from the abdominal wall of a missionary home on leave from West Africa. The adult worm is seen surrounded by multinucleate macrophages in the centre of a granuloma. *(H&E×13)*

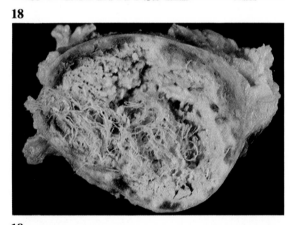

17   Onchocercoma (4410) Section of a skin nodule from a young boy recently returned from West Africa. On the left the adult worm containing microfilaria is seen lying in a track with inflammatory exudate and multinucleate macrophages. On the right, parts of two microfilaria are seen in the granulation tissue in which eosinophil polymorphonuclear leucocytes were not conspicuous. *(H&E×53; H&E×83)*

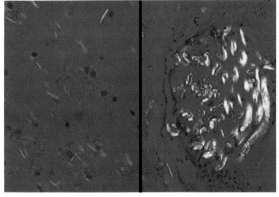

18   Foreign body (gauze swab) in a nephrectomy scar (4410) The lump measured 7×5×4cm and the cut surface shows thick pultaceous yellow-brown material and stranded fabric surrounded by a fibrotic wall up to 9mm thick.

19   Foreign body in a nephrectomy scar (4410) Sections of the stranded fabric viewed with polarising microscope and first order red compensator. The area on the right shows intact double-stranded cotton fibres, while on the left they have been broken into small pieces and ingested by macrophages. *(H&E×133 polarised and first order red compensator)*

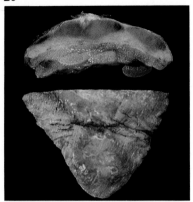

20 **Tattoo granuloma** (4410) on the forearm of a 50-year-old woman. The granulomatous reaction is related to the red pigment (mercury containing).

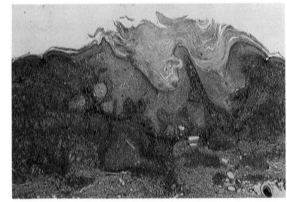

21 **Tattoo granuloma** (4410) Section shows very dense chronic inflammatory cell infiltrate with lymphoid cells, in follicles showing germinal centres, sarcoid granulomatous lesions and foreign-body giant-cell reaction. The overlying squamous epithelium shows marked acanthotic hyperplasia. *(H&E×3.5)*

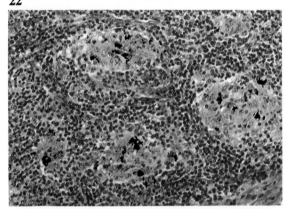

22 **Tattoo granuloma** (4410) Section shows massive lymphocytic infiltrate and aggregates of macrophages with ingested pigment. Plasma cells and eosinophil polymorphonuclear leucocytes are also present in the infiltrate. *(H&E×83)*

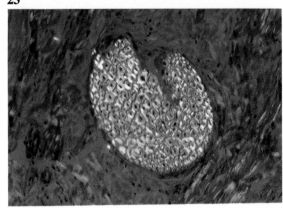

23 **Foreign body in skin** (4410) Section viewed with partially polarised light shows splinter of wood in transverse section with phagocytes applied to its periphery. *(H&E×83)*

24 Perianal fistula (4470) Section of the wall showing tuberculoid granulomatous lesions with numerous Langhans' type giant cells. Alcohol acid-fast bacilli (AAFB) were present in the Ziehl-Neelsen stained section and grown successfully on a Lowensteen-Jensen egg plate from exudate taken from the lesion. The patient was a young Asian immigrant. *(H&E × 33)*

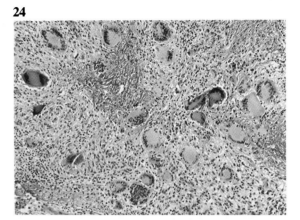

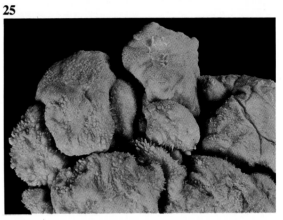

25 Tuberculosis cutis (4470) Photograph showing skin removed from dorsal surface of toes showing warty surface. For 10 years the patient had accepted increasing lymphoedema of lower leg and foot: when nodules appeared on the skin of the thigh a biopsy was taken and showed tuberculoid granulomata in which a single AAFB was identified. Eventually Mycobacterium tuberculosis was isolated on culture. The histological appearance of the illustrated lesion removed by a plastic surgeon was essentially non-specific chronic inflammation with gross oedema and fibrosis, with papillomatosis acanthosis and hyperkeratosis.

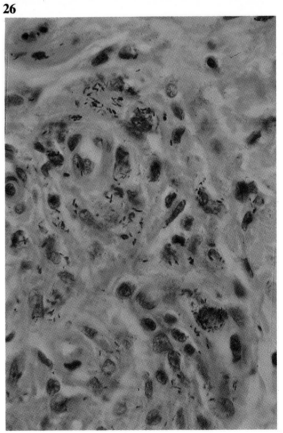

26 Leprosy (4470) Section of a skin nodule from a 26-year-old immigrant who had lived in Dundee for four years. The clinical diagnosis was nodular leprosy. Photomicrograph of the biopsy shows large numbers of acid-fast bacilli (Mycobacterium lepra) lying free and within macrophages (lepra cells). *(Modified Ziehl-Neelsen × 450)*

27

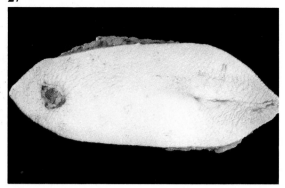

27 Pilonidal sinus (4634) Specimen shows, near one end, granulation tissue forming a swelling around one opening, while at the other end hairs protrude from a slit-like opening with scarred skin around it.

28

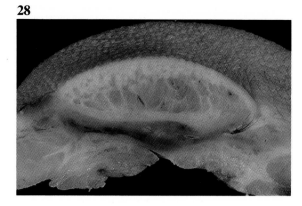

28 Pilonidal sinus (4634) A longitudinal section through the two orifices reveals a chronically inflamed sinus track going deeply almost to the plane of excision. Hairs are seen projecting from the orifice on the right.

29

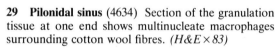

29 Pilonidal sinus (4634) Section of the granulation tissue at one end shows multinucleate macrophages surrounding cotton wool fibres. *(H&E × 83)*

30

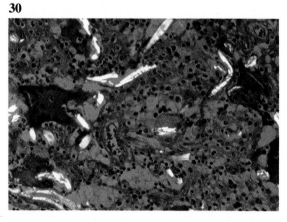

30 Pilonidal sinus (4634) Same section as **29** viewed with polarising microscope with partially polarised light. The cotton fibres appear as twisted, strongly birefringent double strands. *(H&E × 83: partially polarised)*

31

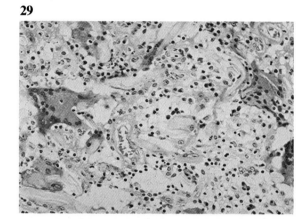

31 Pilonidal sinus (4634) Same section as **29** viewed with polarising microscope with full polarised light and first order red compensator. The fibres appear yellow or blue according to how they lie in relation to the compensator plate. *(H&E × 83: polarised with first order red compensator)*

32

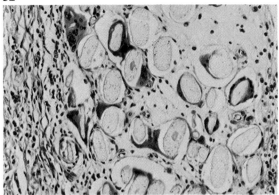

32 Pilonidal sinus (4634) Section shows numerous hair shafts lying among granulation tissue and surrounded by multinucleate giant cells (macrophages). *(H&E×83)*

33

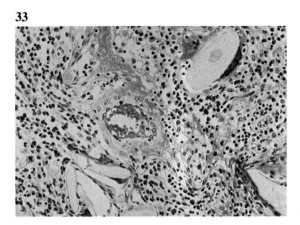

33 Pilonidal sinus (4634) Section shows thick hairs and faintly blue foreign filaments among inflamed granulation tissue containing numerous plasma cells: there are multinucleate macrophages around the hairs. The vessel in the centre of the field shows prominent endothelial nuclei. *(H&E×83)*

34

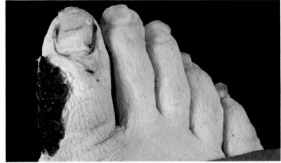

34 Gangrene of hallux (5460) of a 40-year-old diabetic with severe atheroma and medial calcification of arteries in the foot. The discoloured crusted area measures 4 × 3 cm and section shows necrosis and nonspecific chronic inflammation.

35 Tumoral calcinosis (5545) A large (7 × 5 × 2.5 cm) mass from the left shoulder, over the scapula, of a seven-year-old girl known to suffer from dermatomyositis with widespread subcutaneous calcareous deposits (calcinosis universalis). On gross section this mass showed large loculi (from 1 to 3 cm) and narrow clefts containing caseous yellow to white material with hard gritty bits in it. Section showed brisk granulomatous reaction around amorphous calcium phosphate (carbonate apatite) deposits. *(H&E × 133)*

35

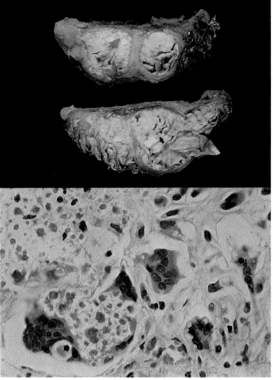

36

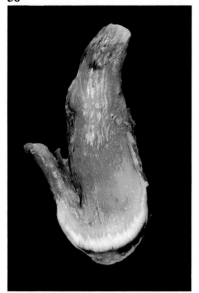

37

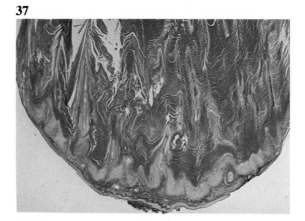

38

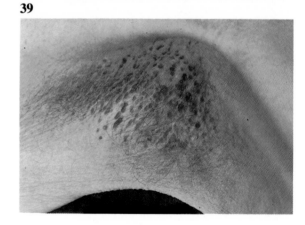

36 Cutaneous horn of scalp (7333) This 3 cm long horn grew at the site of removal, three years earlier, of a similar cutaneous horn on the scalp of an 82-year-old woman. The photograph shows the cut surface with the base clearly demarcated from the subjacent dermis, in keeping with the benign histological pattern of keratinising squamous-cell papilloma.

37 Cutaneous horn (7333) Section shows the base to be keratinising squamous-cell papilloma with fairly dense chronic inflammatory cell infiltrate in the subjacent dermis. The three-year history more or less excludes keratoacanthoma, and there is no histological evidence of malignancy. *(H&E × 35)*

38 Cutaneous horn (7333) Section shows one of the papillary processes covered by acanthotic squamous epithelial cells. Cell bridges are conspicuous and some show nodular thickening (Bizzozero). *(H&E × 133)*

39

39 Acanthosis nigricans of axillary skin (7342) Necropsy photograph from a patient who died of carcinomatosis with oesophageal involvement by a bronchial carcinoma. Most of the pigment in this lesion came out in the fixative (buffered formalin) and histologically there was papillomatosis and only slight acanthosis and melanocytic activity.

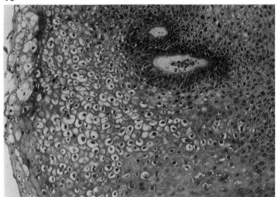

40 Condyloma acuminatum (7344) Section shows squamous-cell papillomatous form with characteristic vacuolation of epithelial cells. *(H&E×53)*

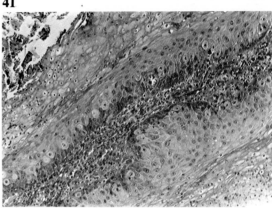

41 Condyloma acuminatum (7344) After treatment for 48 hours with podophyllin. Vacuolated cells are still evident in the outer layers but the striking feature is the apparent interference with dividing cells: mitoses are seen in the suprabasilar layer almost in one layer. *(H&E×53)*

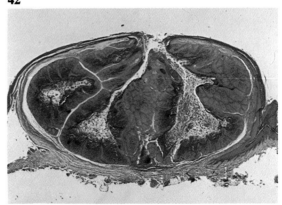

42 Molluscum contagiosum on sole of foot (7347) Section shows flask-shaped cavities containing keratin and molluscum bodies (see **715**). *(H&E×3.5)*

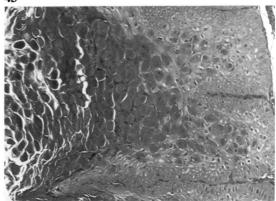

43 Molluscum contagiosum (7347) Section shows molluscum bodies. *(H&E×53)*

44

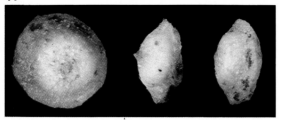

44 Keratoacanthoma (7348) Photograph shows surface view, cut surface and side view. The lesion reached this size (1.5 cm) in three months.

45 Keratoacanthoma (7348) Section showing the typical inverted elephant-bell appearance resulting from keratinisation within bulbous squamous epithelial cell downgrowths. *(H. phloxine tatrazine × 2.5)*

46 Keratoacanthoma (7348) Section shows typical eosinophilia of the squamous epithelial cells with cell bridges (acanthocytes): individual cell dyskeratosis is seen right of centre and some of the nuclei are large with irregular-shaped nucleoli. *(H&E × 83)*

45

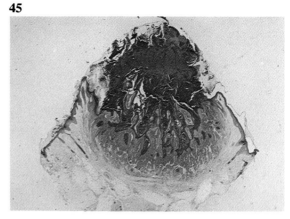

46

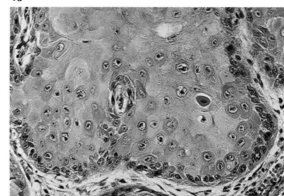

47

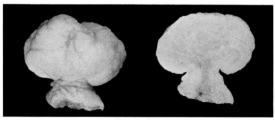

47 Skin tag (7382) Photograph showing side view and cut surface. The fibrofatty connective tissue core is covered with normal skin. The base is 1 cm and the lesion 2 × 1.5 cm.

48 Skin tag (7382) Section shows fibrofatty core with covering of dermis and epidermis. Scattered perivascular and dermal chronic inflammatory cell infiltrate can be seen. *(H&E × 8)*

49 Verruca vulgaris (7353) Section of 'wart' from finger of a child shows squamous papillomatous form and keratinisation at the tips of the papillae: the vessels in these are responsible for the dark dots seen on the surface of a wart if the keratinous layers are shaved off. *(H&E × 5)*

48

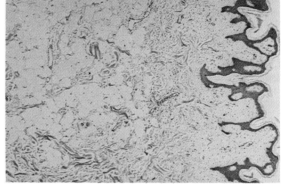

49

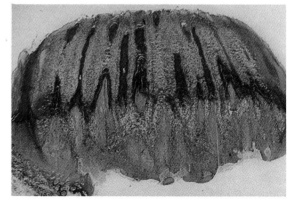

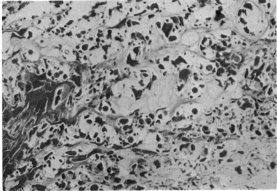

50a   Verruca vulgaris (7382) Section shows deeply basophilic dense nuclei (full of virus) and eosinophilic intracytoplasmic (non-viral) inclusions. *(H&E × 83)*

50b & 50c   Verruca vulgaris (7382) **on thigh of a 15-year-old boy.** Electronmicrograph showing intranuclear virus particles. *(EM × 5,200; EM × 33,000)*

51   Paravaccinia (E 3104) Electronmicrograph showing paravaccinia virus from orf lesion on shepherd's finger. *(EM × 180,000)*

50b

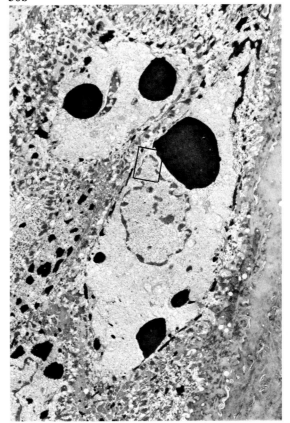

50c

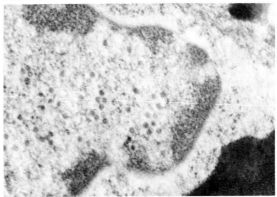

51

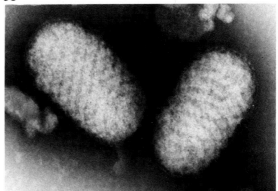

52 Letterer-Siwe disease (7682) (Malignant histiocytosis) Biopsy of papular rash, from two-year-old child also suffering from enlarged lymph nodes, hepatosplenomegaly and lytic lesions in skull and other bones. Section shows infiltration of dermis by large histiocytes with pale staining cytoplasm and vesicular often indented nucleus. The child died soon after the biopsy was taken. *(H&E × 83)*

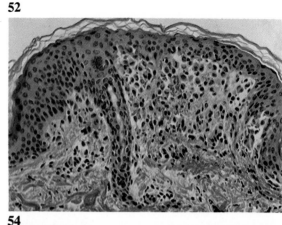

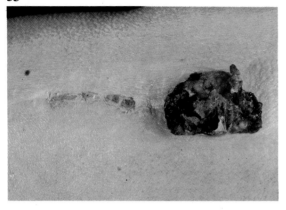

53 Osteosarcoma metastasis (8006) fungating through the incision used to obtain a biopsy some weeks before.

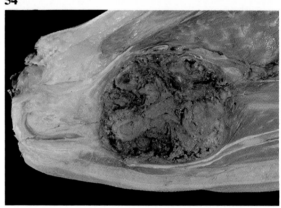

54 Osteosarcoma of femur (8006) Same case as **53**: the proximal part of the amputated limb has been sawn longitudinally through the haemorrhagic neoplastic mass, which was continuous with that fungating through the incision.

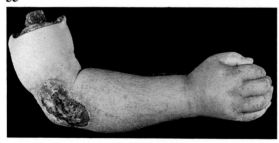

55 Metastatic carcinoma, primary in lung (8016) presenting as an ulcer on the outer aspect of the right elbow, with oedema of the hand.

56 Metastatic carcinoma, primary in lung (8016) Longitudinal section through lesion shows numerous pale nodules of metastatic carcinoma in muscles; bones and joints also show metastases.

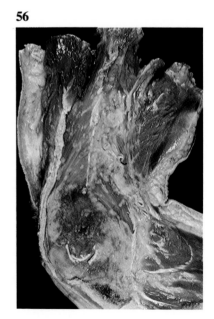

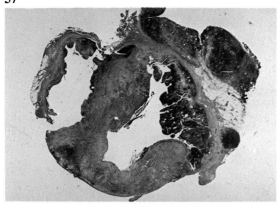

57 Branchial cleft carcinoma (8073) This patient initially presented with a swelling in the neck and biopsy diagnosis was branchial cleft cyst with in situ carcinoma: subsequent recurrent swellings at the same site produced frank carcinoma: no other primary site was detected. *(H&E × 1.5)*

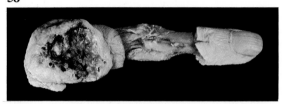

58 Squamous-cell carcinoma of finger (8073) An ovoid (5 × 3.5 cm) raised crusted lesion with central ragged ulcerated area present on the dorsum of the proximal phalanx for one year.

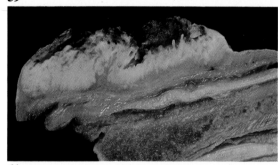

59 Squamous-cell carcinoma of finger (8073) The cut surface shows pale downgrowths of carcinoma into dermis and subcutaneous tissues: the underlying tendon and bone were not involved.

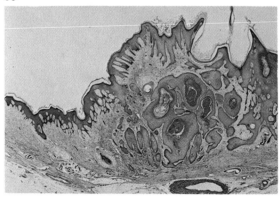

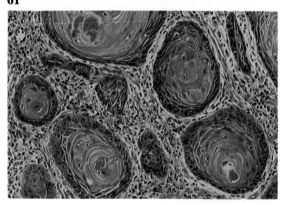

60 Squamous-cell carcinoma of finger (8073) Section shows gradual increase in thickness of the epidermis, hyperplasia giving place to neoplastic squamous-cell downgrowths which show central keratinisation. *(H&E × 3.5)*

61 Squamous-cell carcinoma of finger (8073) Section shows well differentiated squamous-cell islands with conspicuous cell bridges between adjacent squames and central keratinisation (cell nests or epithelial pearls). The intervening stroma shows a mixed cellular infiltrate including both mononuclear and polymorphonuclear leucocytes. *(H&E × 53)*

62

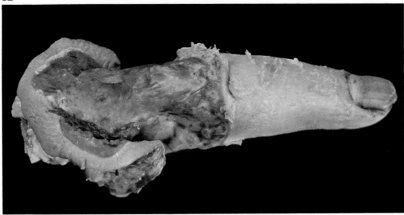

62 Squamous-cell carcinoma of finger (8073) of a 58-year-old man. Biopsy six months earlier was reported as malignant but he ignored requests to attend for further treatment until pain became severe. The specimen is an amputated left middle finger with a near circumferential ulcerated neoplasm 6 cm long and involving all but 1.5 cm of the ulnar palmar aspect. Histologically it reached to within 4 mm of the plane of excision, showed invasion of nerves, arteries and bone: there was calcification in the base of the ulcerated carcinoma.

63

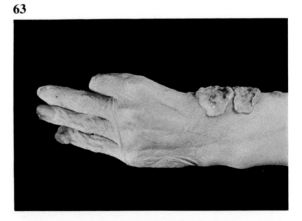

63 Xray induced squamous-cell carcinoma (8073) of the wrist of a radiologist who practised between 1900 and 1927. Part of one finger is missing, nails of the others are deformed.

64

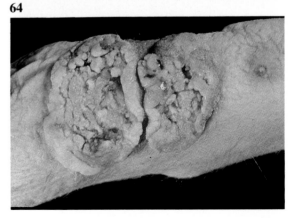

64 Xray induced squamous-cell carcinoma (8073) of wrist; same case as **63**: close up photograph to show two large ulcerated lesions and proximally a smaller one beginning to ulcerate.

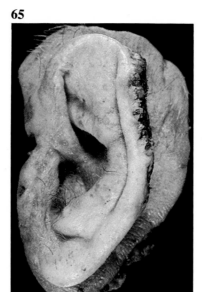

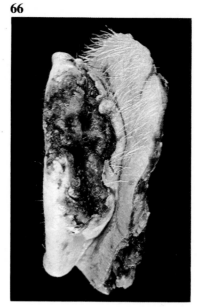

65 **Squamous-cell carcinoma** (8073) of ear from an 81-year-old man with a history of excessive exposure to sun when a soldier in Malaya viewed from the side. It appears to involve quite a small area.

66 **Squamous-cell carcinoma** (8073) of ear; same case as **65** viewed from the back. There is extensive destruction of skin and cartilage.

67

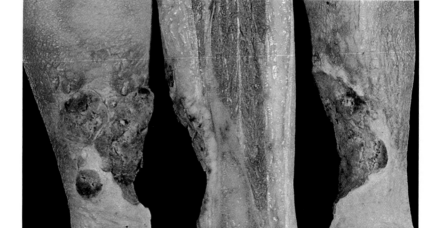

67 **Squamous-cell carcinoma** (8073) of lower leg complicating varicose ulcer, from 82-year-old woman with varicose veins and ulcers for over 30 years. The neoplasm can be seen to have infiltrated deeply down to periosteum.

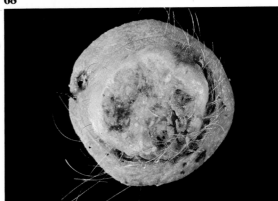

68 **Squamous-cell carcinoma** (8073) of temple: clinically the pearly edge suggested rodent ulcer. The lesion (2.3 cm) was excised and skin graft applied.

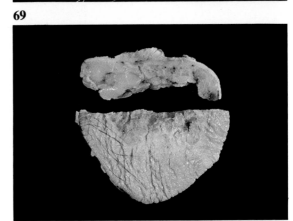

69 **Bowen's disease (intraepidermal carcinoma)** (8082) A skin ellipse from the inner aspect of leg of a 75-year-old woman, shows scaly slightly raised plaque (4 cm). It had been present for several years, slowly enlarging.

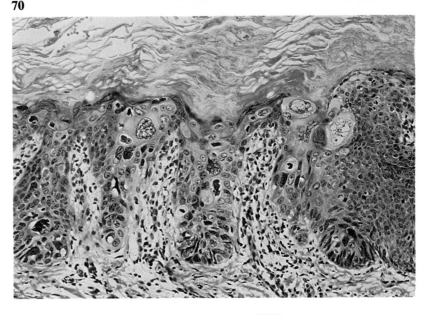

70 **Bowen's disease (intraepidermal carcinoma)** (8082) Section shows hyperkeratosis and irregularly thickened epidermis in which there is disorderly arrangement of cells, many with bizarre giant nuclei, some in mitosis with abnormal forms. There is no invasion. The subjacent stroma shows scattered round-cell infiltrate. *(H&E × 53)*

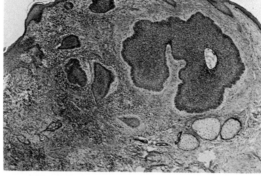

71 Basal-cell carcinoma (rodent ulcer) (8093) Section of the pearly edge of a basal-cell carcinoma excised from the face of a 61-year-old labourer. Darkly staining cell masses show peripheral palisading. *(H&E×13)*

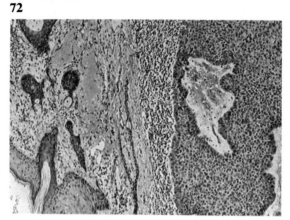

72 Basal-cell carcinoma (8093) A 2cm diameter ulcerated lesion seen from the front. Section shows part of the unaffected epidermis overlying dermis showing actinic elastosis around a tiny basal-cell sprout. The main mass of neoplasm shows peripheral palisading of epithelial cells and there is a heavy round-cell infiltrate in the dermis. *(H&E×33)*

73 Basal-cell carcinoma (8093) Higher power of section (**72**) to show uniform round to ovoid nuclei, several mitoses including an abnormal form (top right). *(H&E×133)*

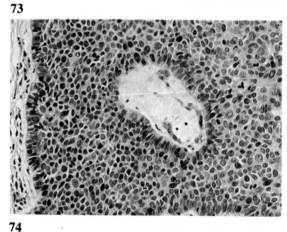

74 Basal-cell carcinoma (8093) Higher power of section (**72**) to show apoptotic bodies caused by shrinkage necrosis. *(H&E×330)*

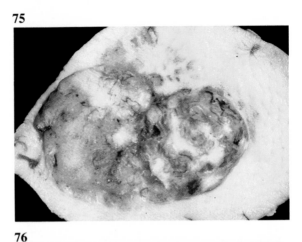

75

75 Basal-cell carcinoma (8093) This lesion (measuring 4.5 × 3 cm) was excised from the middle of the back of a 74-year-old woman. The nodular surface is caused by the presence of cysts. The edge has the characteristic pearly appearance.

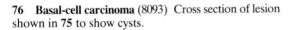

76

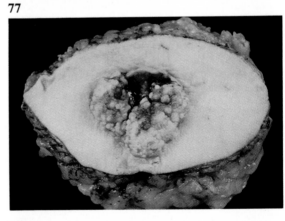

76 Basal-cell carcinoma (8093) Cross section of lesion shown in **75** to show cysts.

77

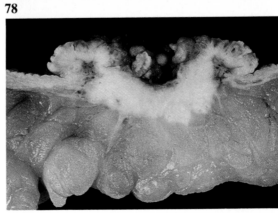

77 Basal-cell carcinoma (8093) from abdominal wall of a 78-year-old woman. It measured 4 × 3.3 cm and was excised with 2 to 3 cm clearance on the clinical diagnosis of squamous-cell carcinoma.

78

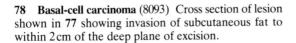

78 Basal-cell carcinoma (8093) Cross section of lesion shown in **77** showing invasion of subcutaneous fat to within 2 cm of the deep plane of excision.

79

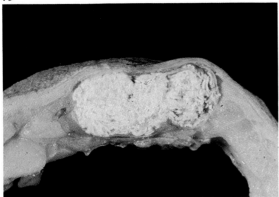

80

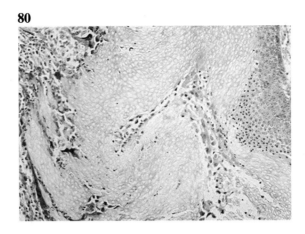

79 Calcifying epithelioma of Malherbe (pilomatrixoma) (8110) This (2.3×2×1.2cm) calcified lesion was situated on the thigh of an 82-year-old man who said that it has been present for only two months. It was fixed to the skin and was thought to be a metastasis so that a wide excision (skin ellipse 7×3.5cm) was done. Histologically it is a classical example of calcifying epithelioma.

80 Calcifying epithelioma of Malherbe (pilomatrixoma) (8110) Section from a lesion on the face of a child; shows basophilic cells, and multinucleate macrophages at the margin of the shadow cells. There was calcification both in stroma and in the necrotic epithelium. *(H&E×33)*

81

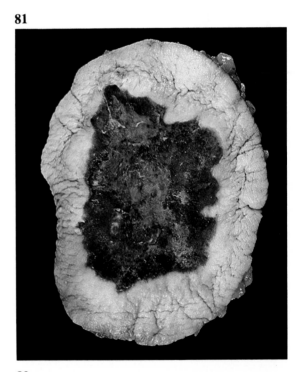

81 Eccrine sweat-gland carcinoma (8403) A large 10×4.5cm ulcerated neoplasm removed from the right leg of a 79-year-old woman. It had enlarged over the preceding two years and was thought clinically to be a squamous-cell carcinoma. Two enlarged nodes from the right groin contained metastases.

82

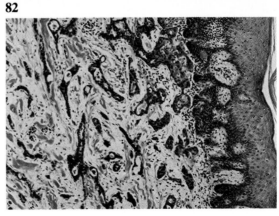

82 Eccrine sweat-gland carcinoma (8403) Section shows tubular glandular and squamous epithelial elements in collagenous stroma. *(H&E×33)*

83

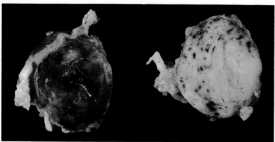

83 Glomus tumour (8710) on proximal phalanx of fifth finger of a 71-year-old man. The (15 × 13 mm) solid mass has a light-brown speckled cut surface. This lesion was associated with paroxysms of pain.

84 Glomus tumour (8710) Section of lesion shown in **83** shows glomus cells in the wall and surrounding vessels in lines and solid mass. *(H&E × 83)*

85 Malignant melanoma (8723) of cheek of a 65-year-old man, present for four months. It was brownish black and hairbearing and 10 mm in diameter.

86 Malignant melanoma of cheek (8723) Section of lesion shown in **85**. It is nodular ulcerated and reaches to the dermosubcutaneous junction. *(H&E × 2)*

87 Malignant melanoma of cheek (8723) Higher power view of section shown in **86**. The neoplasm consists of polyhedral cells, rich in melanin. Mitoses were numerous and included abnormal forms and cells with large eosinophilic nucleoli were common. *(H&E × 83)*

84

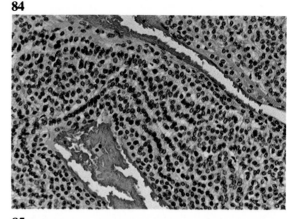

85

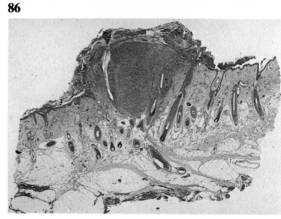

86

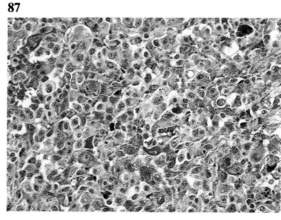

87

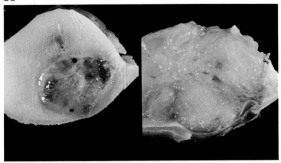

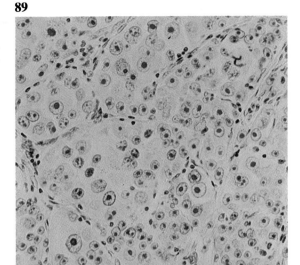

88   Malignant melanoma (8723) of sole of foot from a 69-year-old man. The biopsy specimen was a 4.5 × 2.2 cm skin ellipse with an ulcerated fleshy mass 2.5 × 1.8 × 1.6 cm with pale pink to white cut surface. Cryostat section showed appearances of amelanotic malignant melanoma the polyhedral cells showing nuclei of varied size with prominent nucleoli. When the amputated foot was dissected the lesion was found to be very much more extensive than was thought – it affected an area (5 × 4.5 cm), invaded tendon sheaths and there were metastases in fat several centimetres proximal to the margin of the main mass, and many lymphatics contained neoplasm.

89   Malignant melanoma (8723) (amelanotic). Section showing polyhedral cells with abundant cytoplasm containing little or no pigment and with nuclei showing prominent deeply eosinophilic nucleoli. *(H&E × 83)*

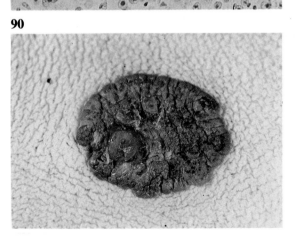

90   Superficial spreading malignant melanoma (8723) (melanocarcinoma-in-situ) from the left buttock of a 56-year-old man, which was present for four years with recent nodule formation. The raised dark-brown plaque (3.5 × 3 cm) shows a lighter brown ovoid nodule near one end. Histologically melanocytes were scattered singly and in clusters throughout the epidermis but also in the upper dermis and forming a nodular lesion.

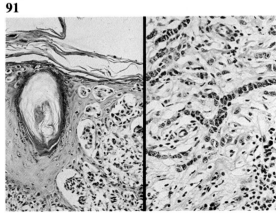

91   Superficially spreading malignant melanoma (8723) Section to show melanocytes within the epidermis with some being shed with stratum corneum and on right infiltrating dermis. *(H&E × 53, × 83)*

92

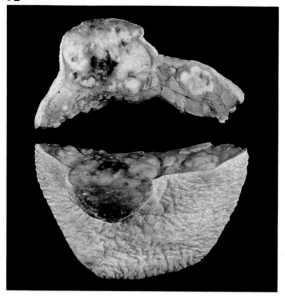

93

94

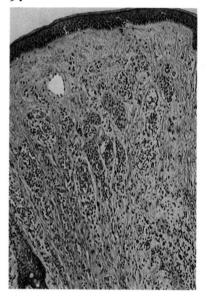

95

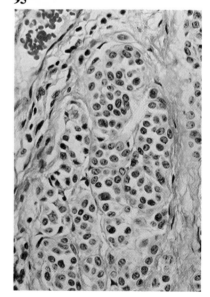

92 Nodular malignant melanoma (8723) from calf of a 72-year-old woman. The main tumour is 4×3.5 cm while the satellite is 1.5×1.0 cm.

93 Melanonaevus (pigmented mole) (8750) Surface view and cross section shows nipple-like projection (10 mm diameter) covered with hairbearing skin. There is light brownish pigmentation of the lesion: the black area (bottom right) is a haematoma.

94 Intradermal melanonaevus (8750) Section of lesion shown in **93** shows packets of naevus cells towards the apex of strands of neural tissue. Surface epithelium shows flattened rete pegs: there are isolated melanocytes in the basal layer but no junctional activity. *(H&E × 33)*

95 Intradermal melanonaevus (8750) Higher power view of section shown in **94** shows packets of naevus cells with small uniformly staining nuclei and pale eosinophilic cytoplasm. *(H&E × 133)*

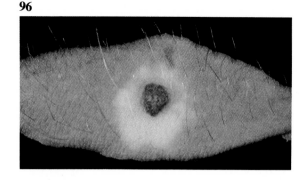

96 Halo naevus (8760) from the forearm of a male nurse present for a year. The specimen is a skin ellipse 4.3 × 1.4 cm with central dark-brown raised lesion 4 × 2.5 mm and halo from 8 to 10 mm wide. Antibodies to malignant melanoma cells are usually demonstrable in the serum of patients with halo naevus.

97 Juvenile melanoma (8770) from the forearm of a 14-year-old boy: clinically the 8 mm purplish nodular lesion was thought to be an angioma. Histologically it shows typical appearances of juvenile melanoma: a compound melanonaevus with junctional activity, telangiectasis, nests of both spindle and epithelioid cells and giant cells. *(H&E × 53)* **97**

98

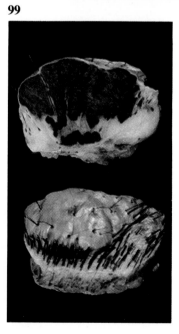

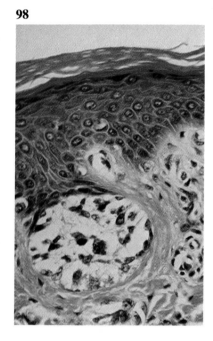

99

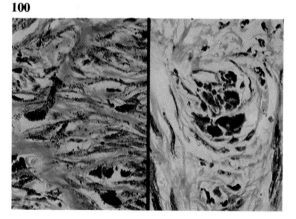

99 Blue naevus of scalp (8780) present since birth from a 26-year-old woman. Surface view shows dome-shaped swelling (3 × 2 cm) slate-blue colour with smooth surface on which some follicle openings are seen to contain tufts of hair. The cut surface is black, as a result of the abundant melanin.

100 Blue naevus of scalp (8780) Sections to show masses of dendritic melanocytes and polyhedral melanophores among collagenous stroma without evidence of malignancy. *(H&E × 133)*

98 Juvenile melanoma (8770) Higher power of section shown in **97** to show cellular pleomorphism in a focus of junctional activity. *(H&E × 133)*

100

101 Sclerosing haemangioma (8830) (dermato-fibroma or histiocytoma). A raised (15 × 10 mm) yellow-ish plaque on the medial aspect of left calf was thought clinically to be an 'epithelioma' and excised with a (9 × 2.5 cm) skin ellipse. The cut surface (left) is cream-coloured with brown areas. When treated with Sudan IV (middle) much of the lesion stains red and with Perls' stain (right) a strong prussian-blue reaction is obtained. Histologically the lesion was reported as a sclerosing haemangioma.

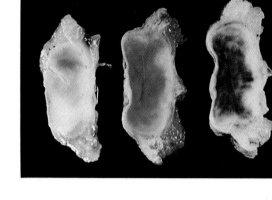

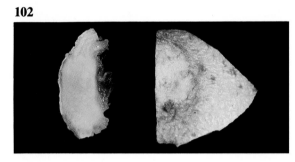

102 Histiocytoma (8830) from the left ankle of a 56-year-old man had slowly enlarged to 15 × 12 mm. It is a raised plaque with distinct yellow cut surface. Cryostat section showed abundant lipid, both neutral fat and cholesterol esters. The lesion was reported as histio-cytoma variant of dermatofibroma.

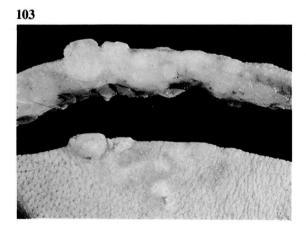

103 Dermatofibrosarcoma protuberans (8833) from the shoulder of a 47-year-old boilerman. It had been present for many years but recent increasing nodularity with ulceration caused him to seek advice. A 12 cm circular piece of skin with nodules (from 2 mm to 2 cm) with pink to white cut surface. The neoplasm replaces dermis and infiltrates the subcutaneous fat for a variable depth.

104 Dermatofibrosarcoma protuberans (8833) Section of a lesion shown in **103** to show characteristic storiform pattern. *(H&E × 53)*

105

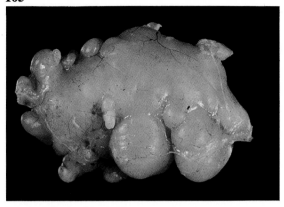

106

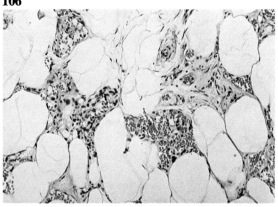

105 Lipoma from forearm (8850) of a 76-year-old woman: she had two other lipomas on the elbow. The mass is lobulated and measures 5×3×3cm: its cut surface shows fat lobules most of them yellow but a few showing flecks of red.

106 Lipoma with angiomatous foci (8850) Section of lesion shown in **105** shows mature adipose tissue cells separated by dilated capillaries: occasional nuclei are large but there was no mitotic activity or evidence of malignancy. *(H&E × 53)*

107 Lipoma with necrosis and calcification (8850) A 5 × 4 × 2.5 cm lobulated fatty mass from the left forearm of a 52-year-old man with multiple lipomata on both arms and legs. This lipoma caused pain.

108 Cavernous haemangioma on face (9120) (necropsy photograph). There were no intracerebral vascular malformations, but the right eye was an artificial one. She died of rupture of an aneurysm of the ascending aorta.

107

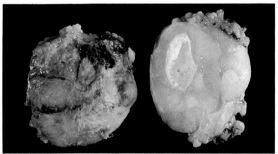

108

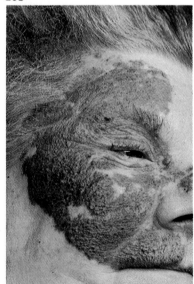

109

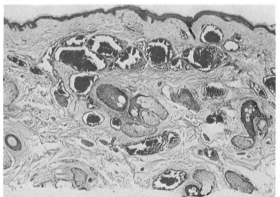

109 Cavernous haemangioma (9120) same case as **108**, showing wide thin-walled blood filled vascular channels in the deeper dermis and subcutaneous tissue. One such channel, right of the centre, shows thrombus in the lumen. The overlying epidermis appears atrophic: the included pilosebaceous follicles appear normal. *(H&E × 13)*

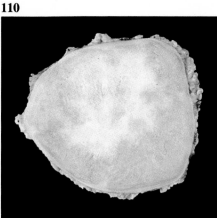

110 Capillary haemangioma (9130) of skin (7 × 6 cm), showing pale areas where there has been spontaneous obliteration of vessels.

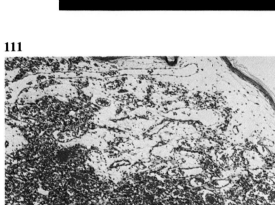

111 Capillary haemangioma (9130) Section shows areas of closely packed capillaries alongside a less vascular area with few capillaries and thin-walled dilated vessels. *(H&E × 33)*

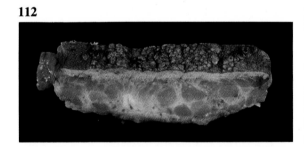

112 Lymphangioma (9170) of skin from a seven-year-old girl presenting with a circumscribed tumour (5 × 6 cm) on anterior abdomen with nodular (up to 5 mm) and vesicular surface. The photograph shows a 1 cm strip taken across the specimen.

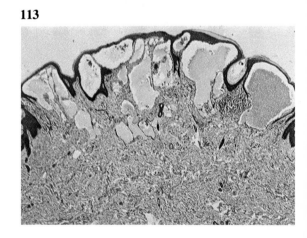

113 Lymphangioma (9170) Same case as **112** showing lymph-containing spaces lined by a single layer of endothelium. They reach very close to the epidermis and connect with deeply placed wide lymphatic channels. *(H&E × 13)*

114

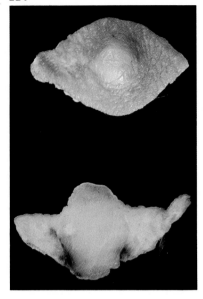

115

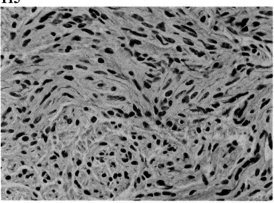

115 **Neurofibroma** (9540) Section of a lesion shown in **114**, stained with Holmes-Alcian method in which axis cylinders appear as black strands among Schwann cells and fibrocytes; connective tissue mucin stains green. *(Holmes-Alcian × 53)*

114 **Neurofibroma** (9540) forming a raised dome (5 mm tall) and excised with a (2.3 × 1.3 cm) skin ellipse (top). On cross-section (bottom) the (12 × 9 × 7 mm) solid tumour with greyish cut surface is seen to reach right up to the epidermis and down to the plane of excision.

116

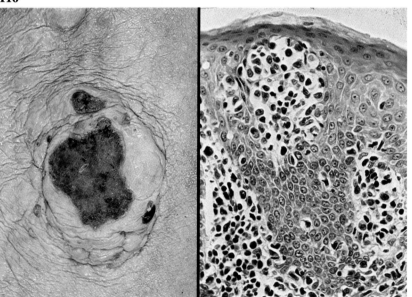

116 **Mycosis fungoides** (9703) in the tumour stage. On left ulcerated (4 cm) lesion: the section shows typical polymorphous infiltrate including large mononuclear cells with hyperchromatic irregularly shaped nuclei in the dermis and also in the epidermis where they form a 'Pautrier abscess': mitoses are always present in the infiltrate – one is included in the Pautrier abscess. *(H&E × 83)*

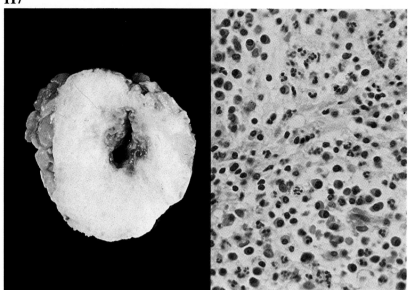

Breast (T04)

117 Breast abscess (4374) from a 37-year-old woman who complained of a tender lump close to the nipple. The specimen is a firm mass ($6 \times 5 \times 4$ cm) of firm white fibrous mastopathic tissue with an abscess cavity (18×10 mm) bounded by reddish brown ragged wall. Histologically the abscess wall consists of granulation tissue in which there are plasma cells, lymphocytes and macrophages some with ingested neutrophil poly-morphonuclear leucocytes. *(H&E × 83)*

118 Mammary fat necrosis (5441) from 79-year-old obese woman who complained of tender lump in right breast for several weeks. The skin over the lesion had been red but was pale by the time the ($7 \times 5 \times 3$ cm) lump was excised. Its cut surface showed two reddish brown opaque areas each about 1 cm in diameter embedded in yellow fatty tissue. Cryostat section confirmed the clinical diagnosis of fat necrosis with brisk granulomatous inflammation. Section stained with Sudan IV to demostrate lipophages: the lipid consists of neutral fat, fatty acid crystals and cholesterol esters. *(Sudan IV × 133)*

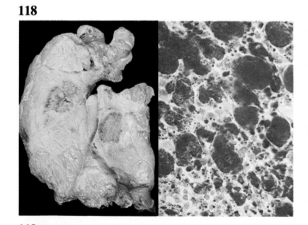

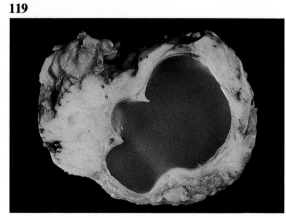

119 Cyst of breast (7631) from 44-year-old woman who complained of a painless lump for several months. The specimen is a ($7 \times 5 \times 5$ cm) mass of mammary tissue, showing mainly fibrous mastopathic changes but with several small cysts as well as a very large (5 cm) unilocular cyst with opalescent yellowish contents and glistening smooth wall. Histologically the cyst lining consisted of flattened and cuboidal cells.

120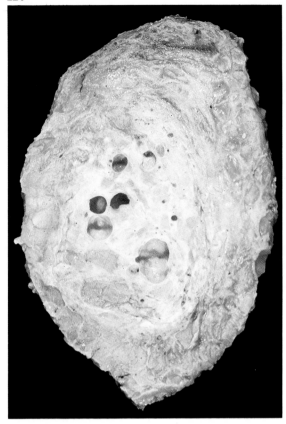

121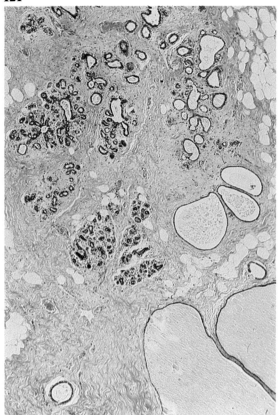

120 Fibrocystic mastopathy (7631) From 47-year-old woman who complained of a tender mass with discharge from the nipple of the right breast. The left breast had been amputated some years earlier for carcinoma. A right mastectomy was done. The cut surface shows cysts of varied size (up to 3 cm diameter) in parenchyma showing white to grey nodular thickening. No evidence of malignancy was found.

121 Fibrocystic disease of breast (7631) Section of lesion shown in **120** shows dilated ducts and cysts, adenosis, and intralobular and interlobular fibrosis. *(H&E × 13)*

122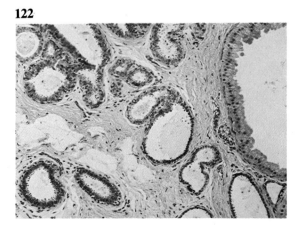

122 Fibrocystic disease of breast (7631) Section of lesion shown in **120** shows ducts with typical double-layered lining, and on the right apocrine metaplasia (pink epithelium). *(H&E × 53)*

123

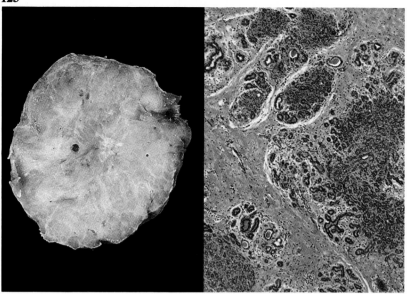

123 Fibrocystic disease of breast (7631) from a 46-year-old woman who complained of a lump in the left breast for two months. It was not enlarging, painless, and there was no discharge from nipple; clinically, radiologically and cytologically (needle aspirate) it was benign. The specimen is a 4.5 cm diameter mass with opaque speckled areas on a white-to-cream coloured cut surface showing one or two blue-domed cysts.

Histologically the appearances are those of a florid mastopathy with marked adenosis and dense desmoplasia (sclerosing adenosis), duct epitheliosis with elastosis, duct obstruction and cyst formation. No evidence of malignancy was seen in sections from blocks including the whole of the cut surface of the specimen. (H&E × 33)

124

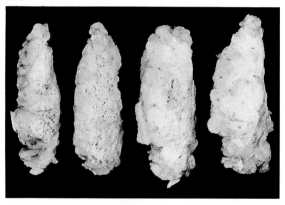

124 Fibrocystic disease of breast (7631) from a young woman who complained of a painful swelling and cancerphobia. The specimen is an amputated right breast partially covered by a skin ellipse (11 × 4 cm) including everted nipple. On serial slices no carcinoma is identified but the breast shows diffuse fibrous mastopathic changes with microcyst formation and duct ectasia. Histologically there was brisk chronic inflammatory cell infiltrate in the stroma among lobules and around ducts and cysts.

125

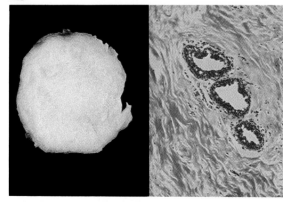

125 Gynaecomastia (7634) in a 15-year-old boy without apparent cause: both breasts were enlarged and a (5 × 5 × 2 cm) disc was removed from each. The cut surface is solid white to grey and histologically shows hyperplasia of duct epithelium and overgrowth of fibrous tissue. (H&E × 53)

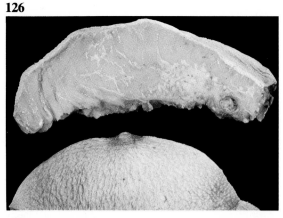

126   Mammary carcinoma (8023) from a 65-year-old woman with backache caused by metastases in spine and pelvis. The specimen is an amputated female breast, partially covered by a skin ellipse (26 × 18cm) showing peau d'orange and everted nipple. On several slices most of one half of the breast is infiltrated by carcinoma, the primary lesion appearing to be a large 7 × 6 × 3.5cm encephaloid carcinoma showing a haemorrhagic nodule at one pole. Histologically the lesion consisted of anaplastic polyhedral cells with little desmoplasia.

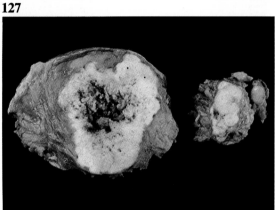

127   Mammary carcinoma (squamous) (8073) from a 69-year-old woman who gave a history of recent enlargement for two months – a clinical diagnosis of cystosarcoma phyllodes was made and mastectomy performed. A huge tumour (maximum diameter 15cm) occupied much of the breast: it showed central necrosis while the peripheral margin was clearly defined though scalloped. The axillary tissues contained numerous enlarged nodes replaced by metastases. Histologically the lesion is a well differentiated squamous-cell carcinoma.

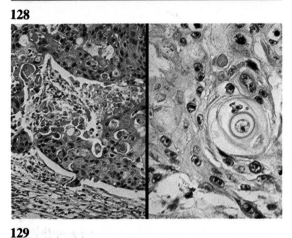

128   Mammary carcinoma (squamous) (8073) Sections of lesion shown in **127**, show well-differentiated squamous-cell carcinoma with scattered lymphoid reaction in stroma, alongside sites of recent invasion. On the right a cell nest shows malignant acanthocytes with cell bridges, some keratinisation and pleomorphic nuclei showing large irregular-shaped nucleoli. *(H&E × 33 × 133)*

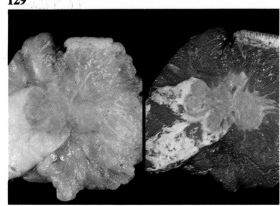

129   Mammary carcinoma (scirrhous) (8143) from a 69-year-old woman who had a negative biopsy three months earlier. The amputated breast contained a (2.8 × 2.2 × 1.4cm) hard tumour which cut like an unripe pear. Its typical cancerous irregular outline is well displayed by treating the specimen with Sudan IV which stains the fat red.

130

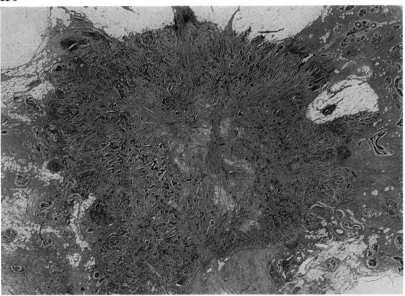

130 Mammary carcinoma (scirrhous) (8143) section of a whole lesion. The patient was a 42-year-old woman with enlarged nodes in the axilla. A cryostat section on a biopsy of breast showed mastopathy with granulomatous reaction but one duct showed changes of intraduct carcinoma. The lymph node showed metastatic anaplastic carcinoma. The mastectomy specimen contained a small (13 mm) scirrhous carcinoma just a few millimetres to one side of the biopsy site, lying deeply and with its margin reaching to within 5 mm of the plane of excision. The section shows the general layout of a scirrhous carcinoma with central zone of acellular, sometimes necrotic or calcified neoplasm, surrounding zone with small packets or rows of polyhedral cells separated by fibrous and elastotic stroma and beyond that more cellular alveolar and intraduct proliferation with infiltration of fat and lymphatics with spread along connective tissue planes. In this lesion a considerable round-cell infiltrate is seen at the periphery of the neoplasm. *(H&E × 2)*

131

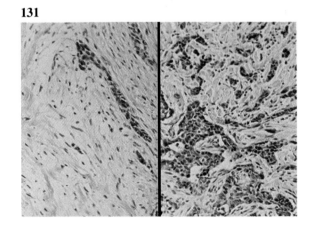

131 Mammary carcinoma (scirrhous) (8143) Section of lesion shown in **130** to show central acellular zone (on left) and more peripherally placed polyhedral cells in columns separated by collagenous stroma. *(H&E × 53)*

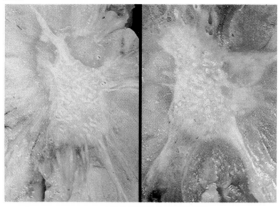

132

132 Mammary carcinoma (scirrhous) (8143) Two examples, each 2 cm diameter, showing typical shape and yellowish-white streaking of cut surface corresponding to areas of elastosis: note also the intensification of yellow pigment in the fat at the edge of the carcinoma.

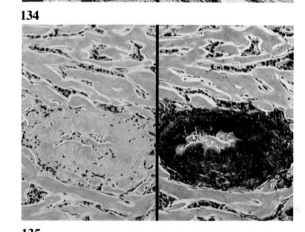

133

133 Mammary carcinoma (scirrhous) (8143) Section of lesion shown in **132** (right) shows periductal elastosis on the left in transverse section, on the right cut longitudinally. *(Elastica H&E × 13)*

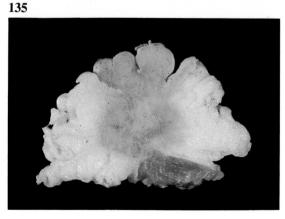

134

134 Mammary carcinoma (scirrhous) (8143) Section of lesion shown in **132** (right) to show periductal elastosis: on the left stained *H&E*, on the right stained Weigert-Sheridan's *Elastica H&E × 53*.

135

135 Carcinoma in male breast (8143) This old man, aged 74, presented with a swollen fungating tumour in his left breast. It had been present for nearly a year. The specimen is a 10 × 3.2 cm skin ellipse bearing nipple, in the form of a 2 cm diameter nodule, which stands 1 cm high and partly covers a (10 × 5 × 2.5 cm) mass of tissue containing a 2 cm irregular scirrhous carcinoma, continuous with the mass in the nipple. Histologically it is of anaplastic polyhedral cell type widely infiltrating the breast, permeating lymphatics and invading to the plane of excision.

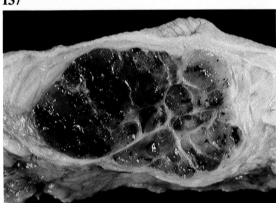

136   **Bilateral mammary carcinoma** (8143) in a 69-year-old woman, who complained of lump in the left breast with indrawn nipple. The lesion (top) is a fairly large (4.5 cm) scirrhous carcinoma. The right breast was found to harbour two lumps – one was taken for biopsy and found to be a (2.2 × 1.6 × 1.2 cm) mucoid carcinoma (site shown by haemorrhage in lower specimen), while quite separately there was a small 14 mm firm carcinoma which showed a varied histology ranging from solid and alveolar with clear cell areas, to adenoid cystic with cribriform patterns.

137   **Mammary carcinoma (mucoid)** (8483) from a woman who for six years was aware of a lump which very slowly increased in size. The specimen is an amputated breast partially covered by a skin ellipse (13 × 6 cm) including indrawn nipple, deep to which there is a large (6 × 4 × 4 cm) mucoid carcinoma.

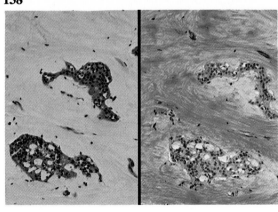

138   **Mammary carcinoma (mucoid)** (8483) Sections of lesion shown in **137** show islands of carcinomatous cells set in a sea of mucin (stained green with Alcian). (*H&E × 53; Alcian, van Gieson × 53*)

139

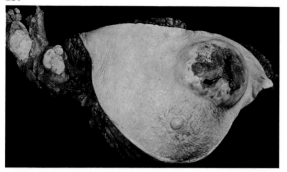

139   Mammary carcinoma (encephaloid (8143) from a woman of 85 with a 2 year history of lump getting bigger and then, 6 weeks ago becoming ulcerated and festering. She was aware of lumps in her axilla. The specimen is an amputated breast partially covered by a skin ellipse including everted nipple. The fungating neoplasm is 8 cm in diameter and forms an irregular ulcer (6 × 4 cm). There are two enlarged nodes in the axillary fat.

140

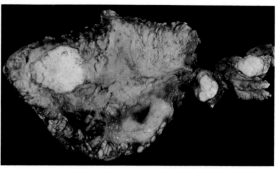

140   Mammary carcinoma (encephaloid) (8143) Cross section of breast and nodes shown in **139**. Note the regular contour and clear cut edge of the large carcinoma with encephaloid cut surface.

141

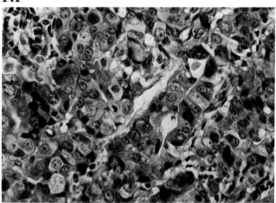

141   Mammary   carcinoma   (encephaloid)   (8143) Section of lesion shown in slides **139** and **140** shows masses of mainly polyhedral cells with very little stroma. In one area (left of centre) there is a suggestion of glandular differentiation with columnar cell formation. Nuclei vary greatly in shape and size. Nucleoli are prominent: there are three cells in mitosis. *(H&E × 113)*

142

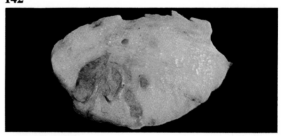

142   Duct papilloma of breast (8500) from a 38-year-old woman complaining of discharge from the nipple. One quadrant contained four dilated ducts in which papilloma is seen.

143

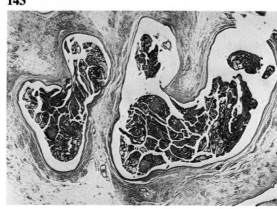

143   Duct papilloma of left breast (8500) from a 29-year-old woman complaining of discharge from the nipple. Section shows intricate papillary processes arising from duct epithelium. No evidence of malignancy was seen. *(× 3.5)*

144 Mammary carcinoma (intraduct) (8502) from a 54-year-old woman, who noticed a dimple in the inner quadrant of her left breast. There were no enlarged nodes in the axilla. The specimen is an amputated breast partially covered by a skin ellipse including a dimpled area deep to which there is a small (7 × 6 mm) scirrhous carcinoma: below it there are dilated ducts filled with creamy material. Sections showed appearances of intraduct carcinoma with infiltration of surrounding breast and accompanying desmoplasia.

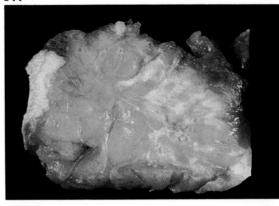

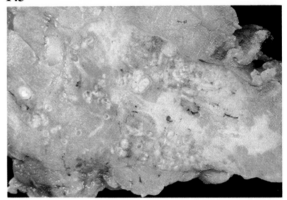

145 Mammary carcinoma (intraduct) (8502) from a 63-year-old woman who complained of a lump in her right breast for some months. The specimen is a skin ellipse 6 × 1 cm partly covering a 8 × 6 cm mass of mammary tissue showing appearances of fibrous mastopathy and intraduct carcinoma: another slice showed small scirrhous carcinoma.

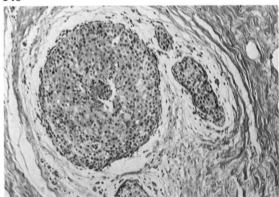

146 Mammary carcinoma (intraduct) (8503) Section of breast from case shown in **151**, shows duct in transverse section with lumen almost filled with neoplasm which appears to be infiltrating into the adjacent stroma. *(× 33)*

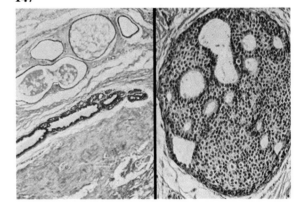

147 Mammary carcinoma (intraduct) (8503) On the left section of breast from **151** showing mammary duct ectasia. On the right section of duct to show cribriform pattern of intraduct carcinoma. *(H&E × 13, × 53)*

148

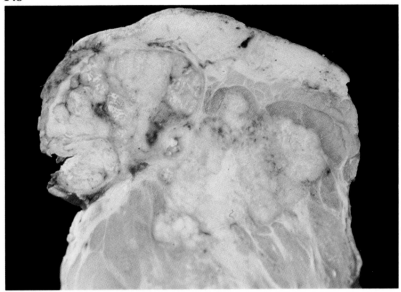

148 Mammary carcinoma (medullary) (8513) from a 70-year-old woman. Needle biopsy unexpectedly showed no malignant cells. The specimen is an amputated breast (volume 1060cm³) partially covered by a skin ellipse (27 × 16cm) including an ulcerated neoplasm in the region of the areola, the nipple having been destroyed. The cut surface shows a bilobed mass (each lobe measuring 8 × 6cm) with distinct edge. Section shows appearance of infiltrating ductal carcinoma of medullary type with very marked lymphoid reaction and prominent plasma-cell component. Lymphatics and veins in the dermis contained metastases.

149

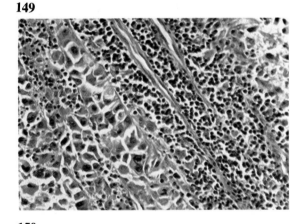

149 Mammary carcinoma (medullary) (8513) Section of lesion shown in **148** to show areas of polyhedral cells arranged in trabeculae and with abundant lymphocytic and plasma cell infiltrate in the scanty stroma. *(H&E × 83)*

150

150 Mammary carcinoma (medullary) (8513) Section of lesion shown in **148** to show metastatic carcinoma in the lumen of veins and lymphatics. *(H&E × 53)*

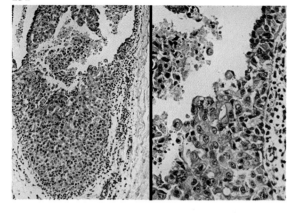

151   **Mammary carcinoma (intraduct)** (8543) Section of breast from 60-year-old woman with Paget's disease of nipple and a large (7×5×3cm) centrally placed infiltrating carcinoma: mammary ducts were dilated and filled with grey-green mucoid material. The section on the left shows transition from the normal to carcinomatous epithelium: on the right higher power shows nuclear hyperchromaticism and pleomorphism and necrotic cells lying free in the lumen. *(H&E × 33, × 83)*

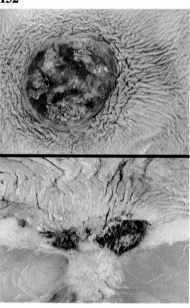

152   **Mammary carcinoma (Paget's)** (8543) On the top, the areola of a 63-year-old woman's left breast amputated for scirrhous carcinoma 3.5cm diameter. It was described as indurated, scaly and tending to exude serous fluid. On the bottom a vertical slice through the nipple of another woman's breast in which a small scirrhous carcinoma lay immediately under the nipple, the site of Paget's disease.

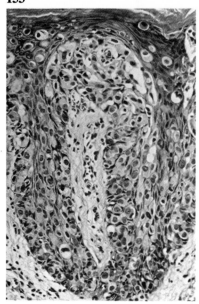

153   **Mammary carcinoma (Paget's)** (8543) Section of nipple from another case of Paget's disease to show large cells with pale cytoplasm and malignant ovoid nuclei singly and in clusters in the epidermis. In this case there was continuity between intraduct carcinoma and the involved nipple. *(H&E × 83)*

48

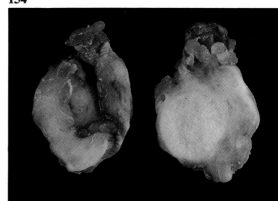

154 Fibroadenoma of breast (9010) Taken from the left breast of a young woman who first noted a lump five months earlier. A (2.5 × 1.5 × 1.2 cm) firm mass was excised and the cut surface shows a near spherical 1 cm mass, clearly demarcated from adjacent fibrous mastopathic breast. There are slits visible among white whorls of fibrous tissue which is translucent. Histologically the appearances were those of intracanalicular fibroadenoma.

155

155 Fibroadenoma of breast (9010) Section on the left is from lesion shown in **154** and shows typical intracanalicular pattern. On the right is a section of a fibroadenoma showing pericanalicular pattern. *(H&E × 33 × 33)*

156

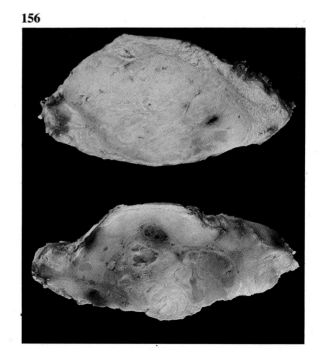

156 Cystosarcoma phyllodes (Brodie's serocystic tumour – giant fibroadenoma) (9020) in a 68-year-old woman who complained of recent (seven weeks) swelling of the left breast. Clinically no enlarged axillary nodes were present and amputation was performed. The specimen is a breast with much of its parenchyma replaced by a lobulated tumour (15 × 8 × 7 cm) with white cut surface generally solid but with clefts and cysts as well as a central gelatinous necrotic area. Histologically the sections showed overgrowth of fibrous stroma with mitotic activity (2 per HP field), and lesser degrees of epithelial proliferation.

157 Granular cell tumour (myoblastoma) (9370) of the breast from a 39-year-old woman who complained of a painless swelling in the right breast. The lesion was of firm consistency and irregular outline and thought to be a small carcinoma but histological section shows it to be a granular cell tumour (myoblastoma). On the left (low power) section shows granular cells in clusters infiltrating fat and fibrous tissue between the breast lobules. On the right (high power) the cells show granular cytoplasm, nuclei which vary in size and staining, with one in mitosis. Such changes are not unusual in this type of tumour which rarely metastasises (see **176**). *(H&E × 13 × 133)*

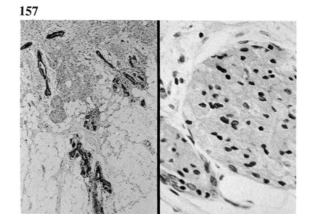

157

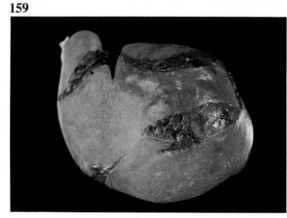

158

158 Chloroma of breast (9933) in a young woman suffering from acute myeloblastic leukaemia. There were several green nodules ranging in size from 0.3 cm to 7 cm.

Spleen (T07)

159 Ruptured spleen (1803) from a 12-year-old boy involved in a road traffic accident and who sustained head, chest and abdominal injuries. The spleen weighs 140 g and measures 11 × 8 × 5 cm. There are three lacerations 5 cm, 7 cm and 11 cm long with large haematomas. Histologically no evidence of any underlying disease was present.

160 Cystinosis (De Toni–Fanconi syndrome) (5500) Section of spleen to show cystine crystals around splenic arteriole: on the left viewed with ordinary light, on the right viewed with polarised light and first order red compensator. *(H&E × 83)*

159

160

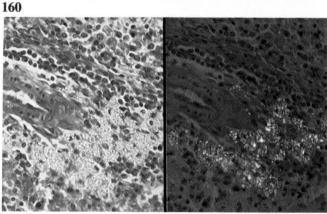

161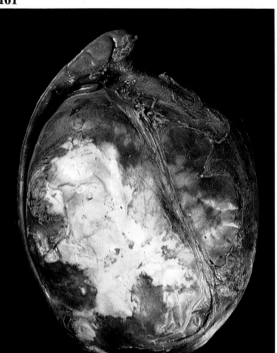

162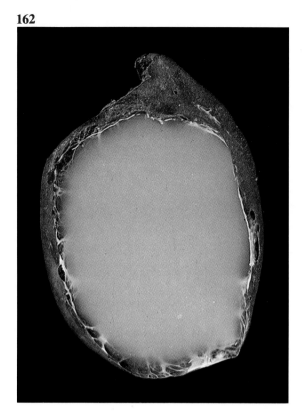

161 Splenic cyst (3540) from a 17-year-old girl who complained of pain in the left side. The specimen weighed 2.5 kilos and showed vascular adhesions and white fibrous plaques on its serosal surface. It was fluctuant and aspiration produced 2 litres of light-brown fluid, rich in cholesterol.

162 Splenic cyst (3540) Same specimen as **161** sectioned to show unilocular cyst with contents, the surrounding splenic tissue shows atrophy of lymphoid tissues: there are dilated blood vessels in one area, and on histological section sinusoids appear prominently.

163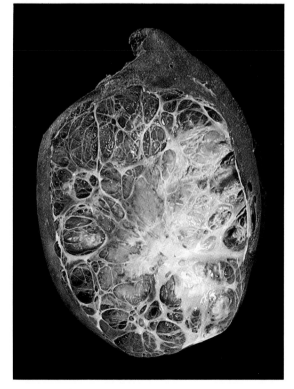

163 Splenic cyst (3540) Same specimen as **161** to show lining; histologically it was lined by squamous cells in 1 to 4 layers.

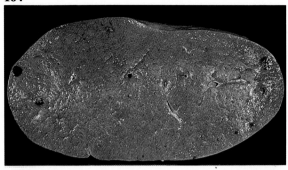

164 Gaucher's disease (glucocerebrosidase deficiency) (7686) in a 47-year-old woman also suffering from a gammopathy. The spleen weighed 1,970g and measured 28 × 14 × 18cm. It showed many adhesions on the serosal surface: the cut surface is a dull salmon-red colour and shows several near spherical haematomas.

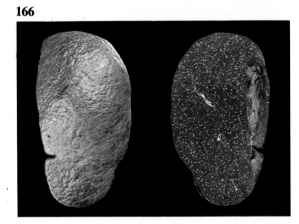

165 Gaucher's disease (7686) Section from lesion shown in **164**. On the left clusters of Gaucher's cells with ground-glass eosinophilic cytoplasm rich in kerasin (a glucose-cerebroside) and acid phosphatase. On the right PAS positive linear parallel striae in the cytoplasm are clearly shown. *(× 133)*

166 Spleen in hereditary spherocytic haemolytic anaemia (7745) from a 6½-year-old girl. The spleen weighed 300g and measured 15 × 9 × 6cm. The cut surface appears dark red and congested with conspicuous lymphoid follicles. Histologically there was congestion of splenic cords, apparently empty sinusoids which contained ghost erythrocytes and had prominent lining cells, some accumulation of siderophages, but no erythrophagy on imprint.

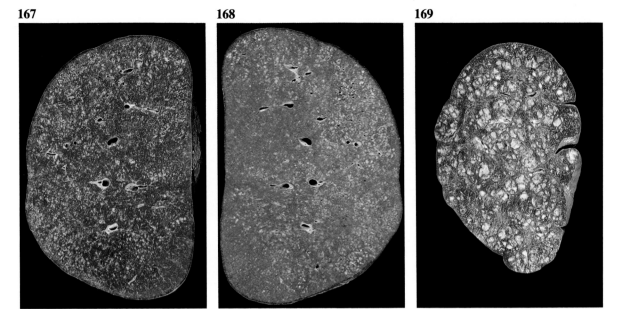

167 Malignant lymphoma (Hodgkin's disease) (9653) of the spleen from a 55-year-old man diagnosed 3 years before as having Hodgkin's disease (mixed cellularity) with enlarged axillary nodes. The spleen weighed 427 g and measured 14 × 10 × 7 cm. The cut surface shows innumerable small pale nodules contrasting with the reddish brown splenic parenchyma giving salami-sausage appearance.

168 Malignant lymphoma (Hodgkin's disease) (9653) of the spleen: same lesion as shown in **167**. Slice of spleen stained with Perls' method: the Hodgkin deposits fail to react, while the parenchyma shows a diffuse prussian-blue reaction.

169 Malignant lymphoma (Hodgkin's disease) (9653) of the spleen: another example showing larger deposits giving an appearance like porphyry or hardbaked toffee.

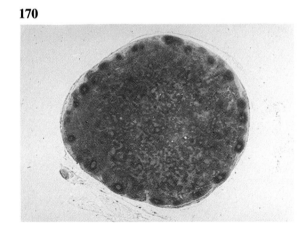

Lymph node (T08)

170 Paratyphoid B lymphadenitis (4200) diagnosed post-operatively after the 15-year-old boy had an appendicectomy and developed post-operative pyrexia with leucopenia. The specimen was one of several enlarged nodes in the ileocaecal angle and was reported as showing a subacute adenitis of unknown cause. The

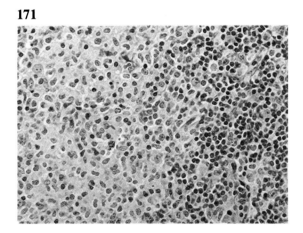

section shows cortical follicles with reactive germinal centres while the medulla contains abundant mature monocytes. *(H&E × 2.5)*

171 Paratyphoid B lymphadenitis (4200) Same lesion as **170**. Section shows, on left, numerous mature monocytes and on the right mainly small lymphocytes: polymorphonuclear leucocytes are virtually absent. *(H&E × 83)*

172 Syphilitic lymphadenitis (4300) from the groin of a 41-year-old lorry driver who complained of swelling in the right groin for two months. He also had penile warts. Clinical diagnosis of femoral hernia was not confirmed at operation when a mass of enlarged nodes was removed. Sections were reported as showing inflammation of the nodes and surrounding tissues and it was suggested that serological tests for syphilis be done. They were strongly positive.

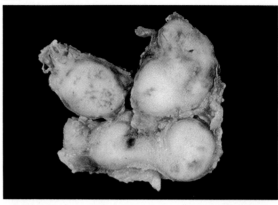

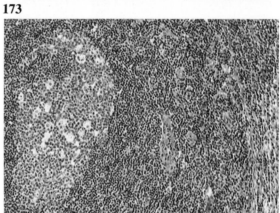

173 Syphilitic lymphadenitis (4300) Section from lesion shown in **172** to show reactive germinal centre and perinodal chronic inflammatory cell infiltrate including plasma cells. *(H&E × 53)*

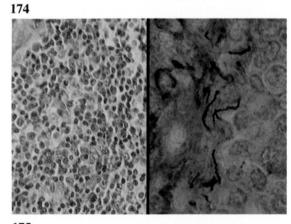

174 Syphilitic lymphadenitis (4300) Sections from a lesion shown in **172**. On the left, section to show mixed inflammatory cell infiltrate with plasma cells, lymphocytes, large monocytes and eosinophils. On the right, a silver-stained section to show Treponema pallidum. *(Bertarelli × 450) (H&E × 133)*

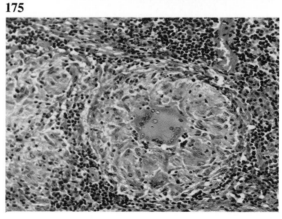

175 Tuberculous lymphadenitis (4470) Section of a cervical lymph node diagnosed as proliferative non-caseating tuberculosis though no AAFB were identified. There is a follicle showing central Langhans' giant-cell with nuclei arranged in horseshoe fashion and surrounded by epithelioid cells, and it contains few lymphocytes: this is sometimes described as a 'naked tubercle', and is often a feature of sarcoidosis. *(H&E × 83)*

176

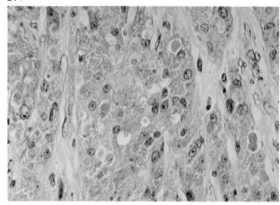

176 Metastatic granular-cell tumour (myoblastoma)
(8006) in nodes in right groin of a 39-year-old woman
who 5 years earlier had had a granular-cell tumour of
the vulva excised. The specimen is a mass of connective
tissue including several lymph nodes, the largest
measuring 3 × 2 cm and showing widespread replacement by solid white neoplasm.

177

177 Metastatic granular-cell tumour (myoblastoma)
(8006) Section of the lesion in **176** showing granular
cells with intracytoplasmic rounded inclusions and
nuclei which vary in size and have prominent nucleoli.
(Red & yellow × 133)

178

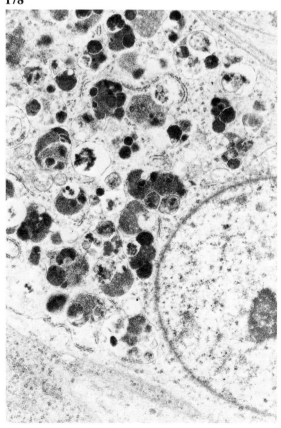

178 Metastatic granular-cell tumour (8006) Electronmicrograph of lesion in **177** showing characteristic
intracytoplasmic   membrane-bound   lysosomes,
generally dense, of irregular shape and coalescing to
form the large granular masses: two other features are
important in diagnosis – enlarged mitochondria and the
presence of a definite external lamina (basement
membrane). *(× 11,000)*

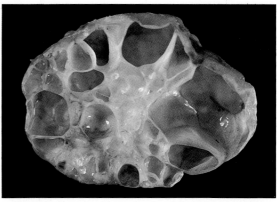

179 Metastatic teratoma (8006) in left cervical node of a 20-year-old man who some months earlier had a teratoma of right testis removed. The specimen is a smooth bosselated mass (4 × 3 × 2 cm): the cut surface shows thin-walled cysts of varied size containing serous and mucinous fluid. Histologically they showed fibro-muscular walls and epithelial lining ranging from columnar mucin-secreting cells to cuboidal and stratified squamous cells, all very well differentiated. The primary lesion had shown well-differentiated and undifferentiated 'embryonal' elements.

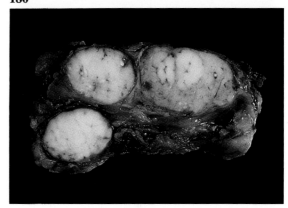

180 Metastatic carcinoma (8016) in axillary lymph nodes in a woman aged 68. The specimen was a (7 × 4 × 3 cm) matted mass of nodes infiltrated by undifferentiated polyhedral-cell carcinoma. The primary was a small scirrhous carcinoma in the ipsilateral breast.

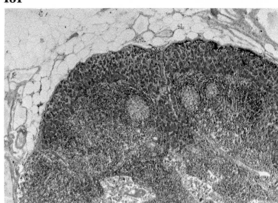

181 Metastatic carcinoma (8016) in left supra-clavicular lymph node from a patient with a signet-ring carcinoma of stomach. The section shows lymph sinuses packed with mucin-secreting metastases stained blue-green with Alcian blue. *(Alcian, van Geison × 33)*

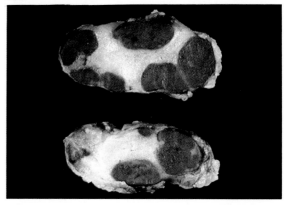

182 Metastatic malignant melanoma (8016) in nodes in the right groin from an 88-year-old man with a tiny (3 mm) pigmented lesion (**185**) on the sole of his right foot.

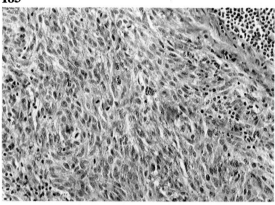

183 Metastatic malignant melanoma (8016) in node. A section from a lesion shown in **182** shows pigment containing spindle and polyhedral cells, with much mitotic activity. *(H&E × 83)*

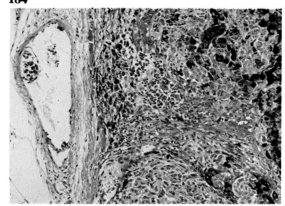

184 Metastatic malignant melanoma (8016) in node. A section from a lesion shown in **183**; metastases in lymphatic and peripheral sinus are visible. *(H&E × 83)*

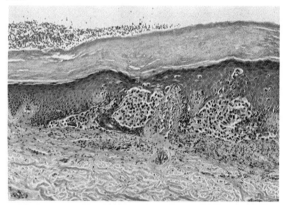

185 Malignant melanoma (8723) from the sole of a foot of 88-year-old man. It was only 3 mm in size but enlarged nodes were present with metastases in the groin (see **182**). No other primary tumour was identified. *(H&E × 33)*

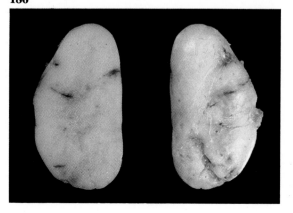

186 Malignant lymphoma (9643) of a cervical lymph node (diffuse histiocytic lymphoma – reticulum cell sarcoma) from a 71-year-old man with generalised lymph node enlargement for a few weeks; he had no other symptoms. The nodes were firm, not tender and mobile. The specimen is an ovoid mass (3 × 2 × 1.5 cm) with uniform homogeneous pink-grey cut surface. The histological report stated complete replacement of architecture by sheets of malignant cells with variable amount of eosinophilic cytoplasm and quite large nuclei, with prominent nucleoli and with many mitoses.

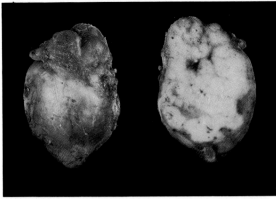

187 Malignant lymphoma (Hodgkin's) (9653) in neck nodes of 21-year-old man with history of three weeks painless enlargement. The specimen is a large ($3 \times 2 \times 1.8$cm) discrete rubbery node with pale lobulated cut surface showing irregular yellow and brown areas of necrosis. Histologically the architecture of the node was reported as showing diffuse obliteration by Hodgkin's lymphoma of mixed cellularity, there being lymphocytes, occasional Reed-Sternberg cells, many mononuclear cells (reticulum cells and lacunar cells) and few eosinophil and neutrophil polymorphonuclear leucocytes.

188

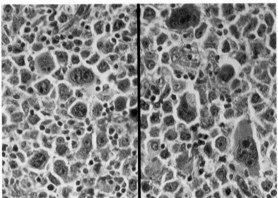

188 Malignant lymphoma (Hodgkin's sarcoma) (9653) A section of node in the lower cervical chain of a 51-year-old man with four months history of enlarged nodes on both sides of the neck and in axillae. The specimen was a firm mass ($2 \times 1.5 \times 1$cm) with fish-flesh-like cut surface. On section the normal architecture of the node is totally obliterated by sarcomatous neoplasm in which (on left) mirror-image cells, and (on right) bizarre giant cells are prominent. (*H&E $\times$ 133*)

189

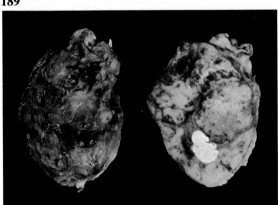

189 Burkitt-like lymphoma (9753) in axillary nodes from a 13-year-old Scots boy, who had never been abroad. He had two weeks history of a firm mass in the axilla. The specimen is a ($10 \times 7 \times 5$cm) lobulated mass with grey-pink cut surface with a large (3cm) calcified white area towards one pole. Cryostat section was reported as lymphoma of uncertain type.

190

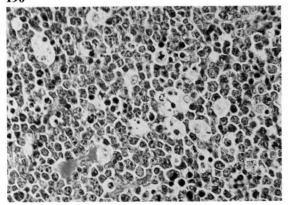

190 Burkitt-like lymphoma (9753) in axillary nodes. Section from **189**. Sheets of lymphoblasts are visible among which are large macrophages containing granular debris, giving the so-called 'starry sky' appearance. E-B virus was not detected on electronmicroscopy of this specimen. (*H&E $\times$ 133*)

2 Locomotor system

Bone and joint (T11 and 12)

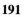
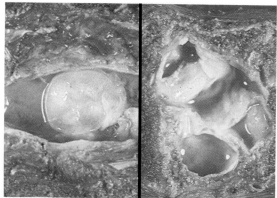

191 Hydatid cysts (3540) in the spinal canal and adjacent thoracic vertebral body of a 66-year-old man. He had had several laminectomies to relieve pressure on the spinal cord and eventually died of myocardial infarction. The cysts ranged in size from 5 to 20 mm.

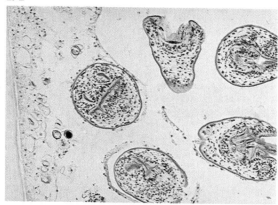

192 Hydatid cysts (3540) The section shows scolices with hooklets. *(H&E × 53)*

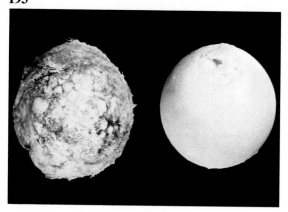

193 Rheumatoid disease of hip joint (4567) A specimen removed at hip-joint replacement for rheumatoid arthritis complicated by osteoarthritis. A head of femur from a control is shown for comparison. The articular cartilage of the head shows irregular erosion at the periphery by granulation tissue (pannus), while centrally it shows fissuring with flakes of degenerating cartilage among fibrinous exudate.

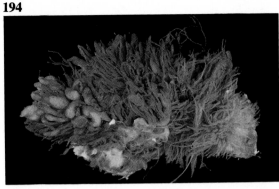

194

194   Pigmented villonodular synovitis (4954) from the left knee of a 36-year-old man. The specimen (200 g) is a solid mass (12 × 9 × 5 cm) with one border shaggy and brown while towards one pole lobules of paler brown to yellow polypoid projections are visible. Sections were reported as showing chronically inflamed fibrous fatty and vascular connective tissue with villous structure in places and extensive deposition of haemosiderin, free and in macrophages including multinucleate forms.

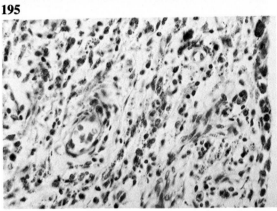

195

195   Pigmented villonodular synovitis (4954) A section of lesion shown in **194** to show accumulation of haemosiderin in synovial lining cells and macrophages, and lying free in chronically inflamed vascular connective tissue in which scattered plasma cells can be seen. (H&E × 133)

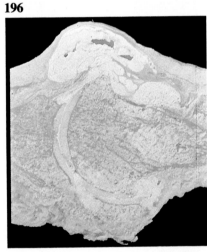

196

196   Gouty tophus (5507) over dorsal aspect of hallux from a 78-year-old housewife who died of myocardial infarction. She was not known to suffer from gout, but both halluces were swollen and white material escaped from small puncta over the interphalangeal joints. The photograph shows a longitudinal slice through one hallux showing the white crystalline sodium urate deposits in the skin, and in periarticular tissue as well as in the joint space, in articular cartilage and subjacent marrow.

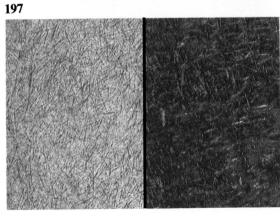

197

197   Gouty crystals (sodium urate) (5507) removed by needle aspiration from the right knee of a 51-year-old man known to have gout. The fluid was turbid and wet preparations showed numerous neutrophil polymorphonuclear leucocytes and masses of needle-shaped crystals which are strongly negatively birefringent. On the left the unstained centrifuge deposit viewed with ordinary light, on the right viewed with polarised light and first order red compensator. (× 83)

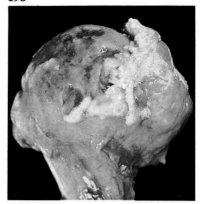

198 Chondrocalcinosis (pseudogout) (5541) affecting the humeral head of an elderly woman who died of ischaemic heart disease. Both knee joints were also similarly affected by the deposition of calcium pyrophosphate producing white encrustation of ligaments and cartilage. The articular surface of humerus also shows severe osteoarthritic changes.

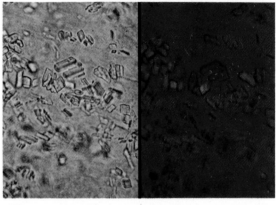

199 Chondrocalcinosis (pseudogout) (5541) Calcium pyrophosphate crystals removed by needle aspiration from the left knee joint of a 93-year-old with a history of swollen left knee for two weeks. Three months earlier the right knee had become swollen and inflamed and radiography showed radiopacities within the joint cavity. The fluid was turbid and contained many leucocytes and numerous rhomboid positively birefringent crystals, both intracellular and lying free. On the left, unstained preparation of coagulum from synovial fluid viewed with ordinary light. On the right, same field viewed with polarising light and first order red compensator plate. *(×330)*

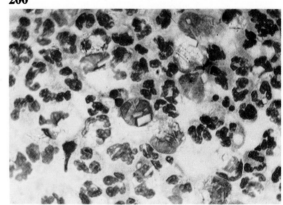

200 Chondrocalcinosis (pseudogout) (5541) Giemsa-stained preparation of knee joint aspirate from another case to show intracellular rhomboid crystals of calcium pyrophosphate. *(Giemsa×133)*

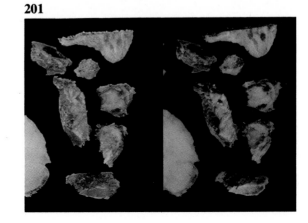

201 Tetracycline discoloration (5500) of the skull from a 34-year-old man. At craniotomy, to remove a neurilemmoma, the neurosurgeon noted that the temporal bone appeared yellow. The fragments of bone appeared normal when examined histologically, but showed yellow fluorescence when examined with ultraviolet light.

202

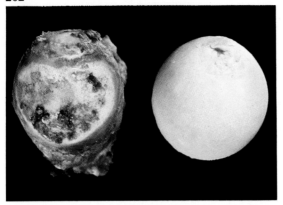

203

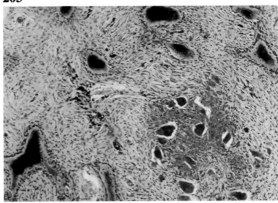

202 Osteoarthritis of hip joint (5023) A specimen removed at hip-joint replacement for osteoarthritis. A femur head from a control is shown for comparison. The articular cartilage of the upper part of the head is completely eroded exposing the bone; in places there are pits where there has been collapse over small cystic areas in the bone.

203 Osteitis fibrosa cystica (7644) in a 54-year-old woman with parathyroid carcinoma (same case as **699**). Undecalcified section of cystic lesion in the femur to show fibrous replacement of bone, focal haemorrhage with accumulation of multinucleate giant cells as well as siderophages. Remaining trabeculae show wide osteoid seams. *(von Kossa H&E × 33)*

204 Fibrosarcoma of the femur (8823) occurring in a young man several years after treatment by curettage of a cystic lesion which caused difficulty in diagnosis – whether a giant cell tumour of bone (osteoclastoma) or an aneurysmal bone cyst. The specimen was an above-knee amputation and the neoplasm was eccentrically situated, 10cm diameter, and had penetrated the thinned cortical bone to invade muscles.

204

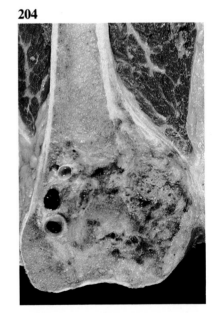

205

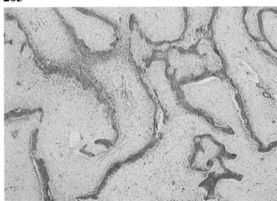

205 Fibrous dysplasia of the femur (7651) from a seven-year-old boy with pathological fracture of the upper end. Radiologically there was a radiolucent zone with ground-glass appearance. Curettage before splinting produced gritty pinkish white tissue. Section shows replacement of lamellar bone by fibrous tissue in which woven bone trabeculae are formed often as sickle-shaped or delicate branches. *(H&E × 13)*

206

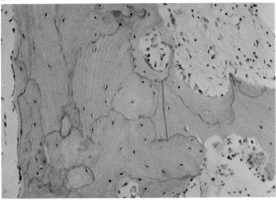

207

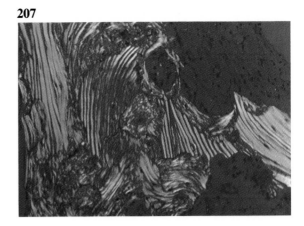

206   Paget's disease of the bone (7657) A section to show mosaic pattern formed by irregular blocks of lamellar and fibrous woven bone, separated by cement lines. Note osteoclastic and osteoblastic activity on right. This patient developed a sarcoma which led to pathological fracture. *(PAS Harris' H × 33)*

207   Paget's disease of the bone (7657) Same section as **206**, viewed with polarised light and first order red compensator.

208   Squamous-cell carcinoma (8016) infiltrating the tibia of a retired minister who had tholed chronic ulcers of his legs for 30 years and more. The changes in the large (22 cm!) circumferential ulcer were those of squamous-cell carcinoma with deep invasion involving the lower end of the tibia. Stains for amyloid were negative.

208

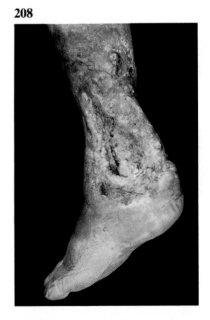

209

209   Squamous-cell carcinoma (8016) infiltrating the tibia. Same lesion as **208** in close-up to show neoplastic involvement of periosteum and bone with local necrosis.

210 Metastatic carcinoma (8016) of the thyroid in the sacrum of a 60-year-old man who ten years earlier had had a total thyroidectomy. The section of sacral tumour showed polyhedral cells, with eosinophilic cytoplasm. Using an immunoperoxidase method it was possible to demonstrate thyroglobulin in the cells. On the left the positive reaction is indicated by the brown colour; on the right the control section has been treated with absorbed reagents, and fails to stain. *(× 133)*

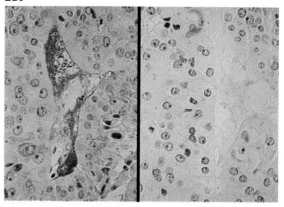

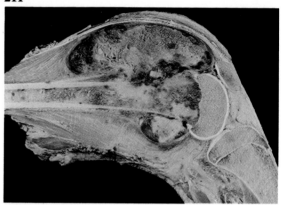

211 Osteosarcoma (9183) of the femur from a 13-year-old girl. The diagnosis was made by open biopsy and within weeks of starting high-voltage radiotherapy the limb became very swollen and painful, requiring amputation of the leg. The photograph shows the haemorrhagic sarcoma involving 12 cm of the lower end of femur with periosteal elevation. *(Codman's triangle)*

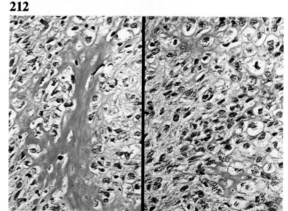

212 Osteosarcoma (9183) of right humerus occurring ten years after radiotherapy for mammary carcinoma of the right breast. Section shows diagnostic new bone formation by the tumour cells: the osteoid takes the form of eosinophil strands. Sections show (left) areas of osteoid and undifferentiated spindle cells, and (right) an area of chondroid differentiation. The latter may be very conspicuous in some osteosarcomas, so that it is important to examine sections from several blocks selected preferably after study of a radiograph of the specimen avoiding the reactive periosteal new bone. *(H&E × 83)*

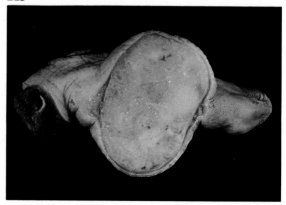

213 Enchondroma (9220) from a 58-year-old man whose little finger had gradually become swollen over several years. The middle phalanx of the finger is replaced by an ovoid swelling (4 × 3 × 3 cm). Its cut surface is bluish white and glassy, like hyaline cartilage.

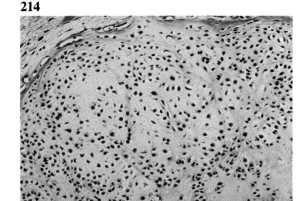

214 Enchondroma of the finger (9220) Same lesion as 213. Section shows lobules of cartilaginous matrix with cartilage cells showing some nuclear pleomorphism, with occasional twinned nuclei but there were only very occasional mitoses. It was reported as an enchondroma for which complete excision should suffice: cartilaginous neoplasms of the fingers rarely metastasise. *(H&E × 53)*

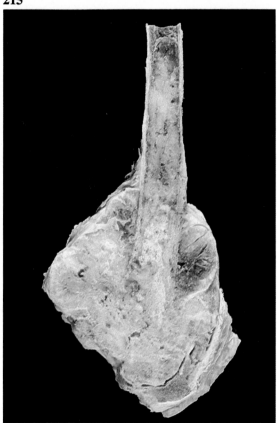

215 Chondrosarcoma (9223) of the femur from a 70-year-old woman who two years before had complained of discomfort in her left knee: an xray had shown, she was told, degenerative changes. Increasing swelling with pain had forced her to seek help. Radiographs showed changes strongly suggestive of chondrosarcoma; this was confirmed by biopsy. Amputation was carried out 26cm above the knee joint leaving 8mm clearance. The distal half of femur shows widespread destruction of cortex with large (4 to 5cm) extraosseous extensions mostly translucent and bluish white though sometimes soft brownish and necrotic. A dense sclerotic zone in the medulla begins several centimetres above the articular cartilage. There were severe osteoarthritic changes in the knee joint.

216 Osteochondroma (9210) of the ileum in a 17-year-old boy who complained of a hard mass in his lower abdomen. An xray taken in his home town had been reported as showing appearances of osteosarcoma, but at operation the lesion was obviously an osteocartilaginous one with, on histological examination, only a minor degree of nuclear pleomorphism, occasional twinning, and virtually no mitotic activity. Despite the benign histological appearances it was felt that the behaviour of any cartilaginous tumour of the ileum was unpredictable and regular follow up was advised, particularly as it was not certain whether complete clearance had been achieved.

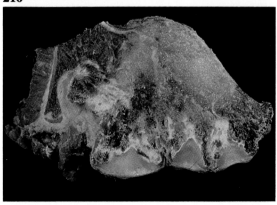

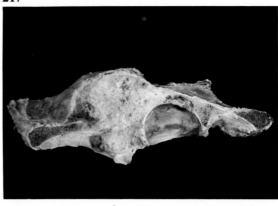

217 Chondrosarcoma (9223) of the ileum in a 62-year-old woman, treated by hindquarter amputation. The specimen consisted of the right leg and most of the right hemipelvis. The plane of resection through the wing of the ileum showed one large (3 cm) and three small (5 mm) transected foci of gelatinous neoplasm. The largest tumour mass measured 6 × 5 cm and it destroyed much of the ileum above the acetabulum and bulged into the iliopsoas: histologically the lesion was a highly cellular chondrosarcoma.

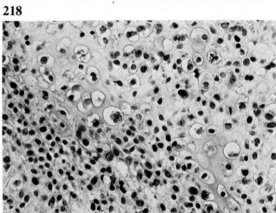

218 Chondrosarcoma (9223) A section to show highly cellular areas with malignant chondroblasts in lacunae and showing nuclear pleomorphism, twinning and mitoses including abnormal forms. *(H&E × 83)*

219 Giant-cell tumour of the bone (osteoclastoma) (9251) from a medial femoral condyle of a 24-year-old woman, who had complained of swelling of the knee for six months. Radiologically there was expansion of the cortex at the lower end of the femur. The specimen was obtained by curettage and consists of irregular pieces of fairly firm tissue ranging in size from 3 × 1.5 cm, to 4 × 3.5 cm, and mainly brown to red with yellow areas and three pieces of pinkish-white periosteal tissue. Section shows vascularised spindle-cell stroma with abundant multinucleate giant cells of osteoblast type, evenly distributed throughout. Mitoses were numerous; in one section of the periosteum a vein showed giant-cell tumour in its lumen.

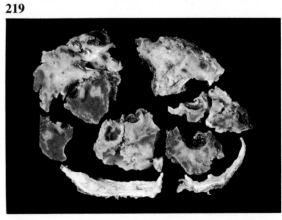

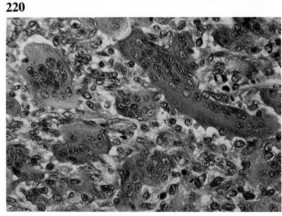

220 Giant-cell tumour of the bone (osteoclastoma) (9251) Section from the lesion shown in **219** shows multinucleate giant cells of varied size, separated by proliferating spindle cells. *(H&E × 133)*

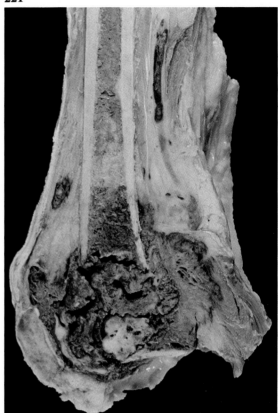

221 Giant-cell tumour of bone (osteoclastoma) (9253) from a 47-year-old woman with destructive lesion at lower end of right femur and pathological fracture. Mid-thigh amputation was done. The leg was markedly swollen and on dissection the lower end of the femur with much of the articular cartilage had been destroyed by soft haemorrhagic neoplasm, which directly invaded the suprapatellar pouch and two major veins in the thigh. Histologically the lesion was reported as a very aggressive malignant giant-cell tumour of bone with invasion of veins.

222

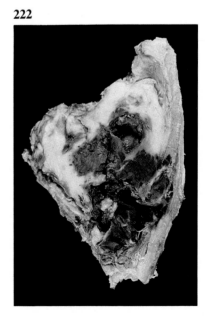

222 Giant-cell tumour of sacrum (9251) from a 39-year-old woman who presented initially with neurological symptoms of L5-S1 sensory loss: nothing abnormal was detected. Eleven months later at vaginal examination a gynaecologist felt a swelling: at laparotomy the true nature of the swelling was not immediately apparent and partial removal led to haemorrhage and subsequent fatal septicaemia. Histologically the lesion was a giant-cell tumour of bone.

223 **Ewing's sarcoma** (9263) of the rib from a nine-year-old girl. The specimen is a 10cm long piece of rib with an 8 × 6 × 4cm smooth mass showing a pink-grey fleshy cut surface. On section it consisted of cells with uniform round nuclei and PAS-positive glycogen-rich cytoplasm, without much reticulin and showing no rosettes. Electronmicrographs showed polyhedral cells rich in glycogen with occasional lipid droplets and poorly developed organelles.

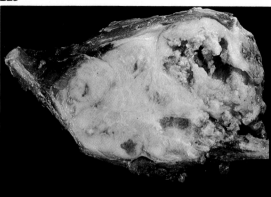

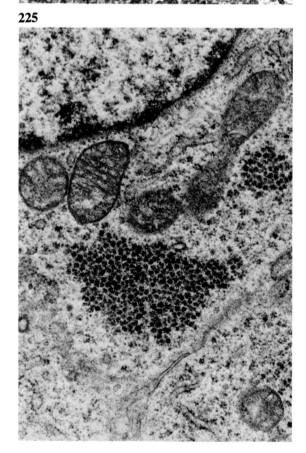

224 **Ewing's sarcoma** (9263) of the rib. A section from the lesion in **223** showing the appearance of a proliferating malignant round-cell tumour. *(H&E × 133)*

225 **Ewing's sarcoma** (9263) of the rib. Electronmicrograph of the lesion in **223** to show intracytoplasmic glycogen. *(× 25,000)*

226 **Ewing's sarcoma** (9263) of the left humerus from a three-year-old girl. The specimen was dissected out from the amputated limb and shows the greatly expanded proximal half with cross section equal to that of the humeral head. The neoplasm had penetrated the cortex over the upper 5cm and infiltrated muscle. The bone was sawn longitudinally showing almost complete replacement of marrow by soft pale rather gelatinous neoplasm. A small 8mm cyst lay in the centre of the distal end. The histological diagnosis offered was round-cell sarcoma: subsequent staining with PAS, and electronmicroscopy confirmed the presence of much glycogen in the cells. The child survived for six months only.

226

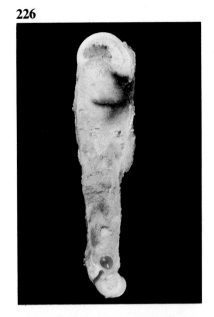

227

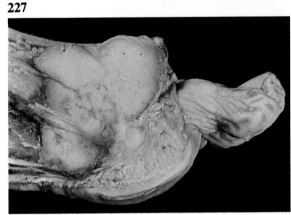

227 **Extra-osseous Ewing's sarcoma** (9263) of the foot from a 24-year-old man with a two-year history of a swelling on the dorsum of his right foot. A biopsy diagnosis of synoviosarcoma was suggested, but continuing survival (after 15 years) in the light of recent interest in glycogen content of Ewing's sarcoma led to re-examination of the material by light and electronmicroscopy confirming the presence of glycogen, thus making Ewing's sarcoma the likely diagnosis. The specimen was an amputated right foot and distal 20cm of leg. The dorsum of foot bore a prominent bulge (6 × 5cm). On dissection a mass (8 × 5 × 5cm) which was lobulated, pale yellowish-white and firm, was exposed spreading from the dorsum between the 2nd and 3rd metatarsals on the sole of the foot: the tendons of extensor digitorum longus to the 2nd and 3rd toes passed through the substance of the mass. Sixteen years after amputation he presented with breathlessness, cough and raised ESR; a pleural biopsy showed metastases with appearances similar to those seen in the original lesion.

228

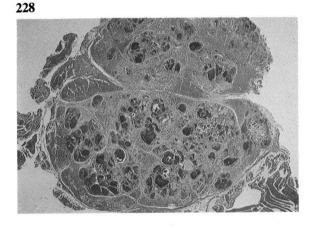

228 **Haemangioma** (9120) in muscle from a 19-year-old girl with a three-year history of feeling a lump in her right thigh. At operation the application of tourniquet caused the swelling (5 × 5cm) to disappear! Eventually the lesion, now measuring only 2 × 1.5 × 1.3cm, was excised with some surrounding muscle. Section showed both capillary and cavernous haemangioma with the vascular spaces filled with blood – some containing organised, partly calcified and ossified thrombus. Large malformed vessels, in keeping with an arteriovenous malformation, were evident. The adjacent muscle showed both degenerative and chronic inflammatory changes. (×2)

Muscle (T13)

229 Myxosarcoma (8843) of muscle of the left thigh from a 77-year-old woman who had a similar lesion removed from the same site two years earlier. The specimen is a (8 × 5 cm) mass of muscle embedded in which there is a gelatinous mass (7 × 4 cm): on section it showed appearances of myxosarcoma similar to the lesion removed earlier.

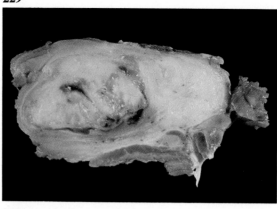

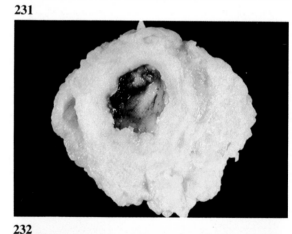

230 Myxosarcoma (8843) of muscle. A section of lesion shown in **229**: on the left stained (H&E) to show sarcomatous stellate cells with pleomorphic nuclei lying in abundant mucinous matrix, which appears green in the section (on right) stained with Alcian blue. (× 53)

Bursa (T16)

231 Prepatellar chronic bursitis (4300) from the right knee of a five-year-old boy. Clinically it was thought to be a lipoma, and had been present for two years. The specimen is a fibrofatty mass (4 × 3.5 × 1.5 cm) in which a 2 cm diameter cavity contains bloodstained fluid. Section showed appearances of a bursa with chronically inflamed synovial lining. In an older female patient such a lesion would qualify as 'housemaid's knee'.

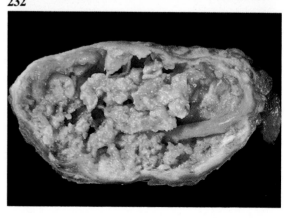

232 Chronic bursitis (4300) from the left elbow of a 55-year-old insurance agent, who complained of a gradually enlarging non-painful lump which he found an inconvenience and unsightly. He had gout. The specimen is a nodular cystic (8 × 5 × 3 cm) mass containing yellow-brown cholesterol-rich fluid. Microscopically the wall is collagenous with granulomatous reaction around cholesterol crystals.

233

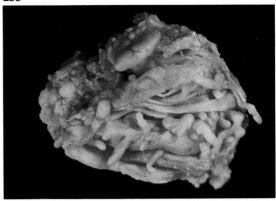

233 Olecranon bursa (5541) from a 57-year-old man. The specimen is an (5 × 3 cm) opened bursa with partly calcified contents. The wall shows pale villous projections as well as bridging bands which histologically are lined with synovium. There was little or no evidence of inflammation.

234

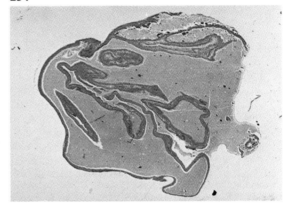

234 Calcareous bursitis (5541) from a young man on dialysis as a result of renal failure. Section of bursa filled with toothpaste-like material. Histologically there is granulomatous reaction around the granules of calcium phosphate complexes (apatite). *(H&E×2)*

235

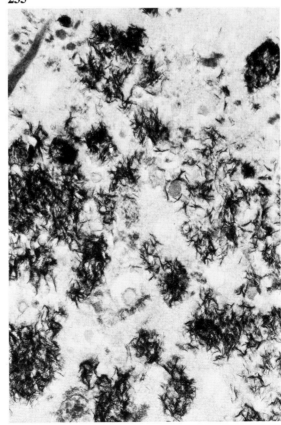

235 Calcareous bursitis (5541) Electronmicrograph of calcareous material from a bursa from another (renal failure) patient on dialysis, to show calcium phosphate (apatite) crystals. *(×17,000)*

Tendon and tendon sheath (T17)

236 Ganglion cyst (3555) from a medial aspect of the right knee from a 43-year-old man. The specimen is a pyriform mass ($4 \times 3 \times 2$ cm) containing glairy fluid. Histologically the fibrous wall showed mucinous degeneration – there was no synovial lining thus distinguishing it from a bursa.

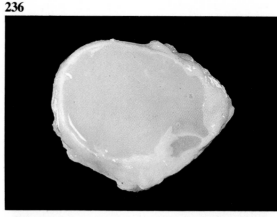

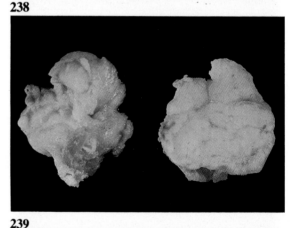

237 Localised nodular tenosynovitis (4953) (benign synovioma or giant-cell tumour of tendon sheath). A swelling on the left index finger of a 41-year-old woman. At operation it was attached to the tendon sheath, was a brown colour and nodular with a groove along one side. It was $4 \times 2 \times 1.5$ cm and histologically showed appearances of localised nodular tenosynovitis, with abundant haemosiderin free and in macrophages.

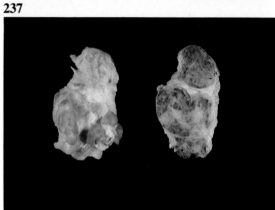

238 Malignant histiocytoma (8803) from the right forearm of a 36-year-old woman with several years history of painless mass recently causing neurological damage to the radial nerve. The specimen is an irregular mass ($4 \times 2 \times 2$ cm) with creamy-yellow lobules separated by white strands. Histologically the main cell type is spindle cell showing pleomorphism and numerous mitoses, some of the aberrant type. Substantial amounts of lipid (including birefringent forms) are demonstrable in histiocytes in frozen sections. Storiform patterns were seen in some areas.

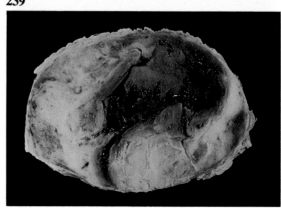

239 Liposarcoma (8853) of the left knee from a 68-year-old man. He complained of a swelling for one year, which became larger and painful recently. The mass ($7 \times 7 \times 4.5$ cm) was attached to the muscle on the medial aspect of the left knee and its cut surface showed red, yellow, orange and white areas, generally soft, in places slimy, with areas of haemorrhage and necrosis. Histologically the neoplasm was variable in appearance, with spindle cells, stellate cells and pleomorphic cells, some containing sudanophilic lipid.

3 Respiratory system

Nose (T21)

240 Rhinophyma (4548) from an 80-year-old man with a history of a slowly enlarging growth on the nose for five years. It was excised as seven pieces ranging in size from 2.5 to 8 cm. The cut surface is pinkish-white to yellow, generally translucent, but with opaque brownish areas. Histologically it consists of oedematous highly vascular connective tissue, showing focal chronic inflammatory cell infiltrate and with prominent sebaceous glands.

241 Nasal polyp (7381) Two of several removed from the nasal cavities and ethmoid sinus of a 61-year-old woman with a long history of allergic rhinitis. The specimen shows two polyps 15 and 20 mm in diameter, each with a narrow stalk, and with oedematous translucent stroma and opaque mucin-containing cysts. Microscopically a mixed chronic inflammatory cell infiltrate included many eosinophils and plasma cells.

242 Giant choanal polyp (7381) from a 16-year-old boy with a history of 'stuffy' nose. The specimen is a bilobed mass 5 cm long and each lobe measuring 2.5 × 2 cm. One lobe is cystic and the other is solid, but markedly oedematous. Sections showed chronic inflammatory cell infiltrate, in which plasma cells and lymphocytes predominated.

240

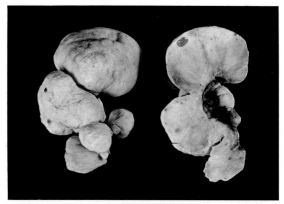

241

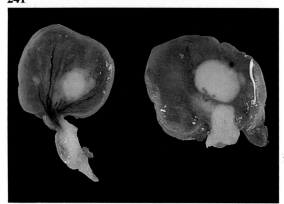

242

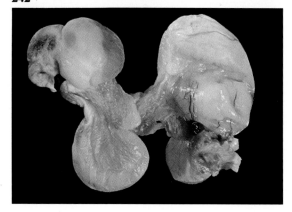

243 Allergic polyps (7381) from the nose of a 35-year-old man with a long history of allergic rhinitis and two previous polypectomies. The sections of the 14 polyps all showed similar appearances: oedematous stroma packed with eosinophil polymorphonuclear leucocytes, several macrophages with ingested eosinophil polymorphonuclear leucocytes and showing Charcot-Leyden crystal development, and sparse plasma cells. *(H&E × 330)*

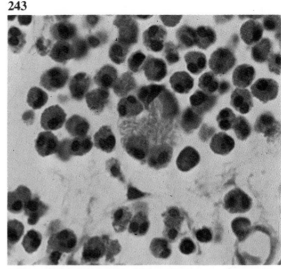

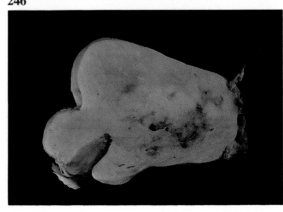

244 Nasal papilloma (8120) recurrence in the nose of 58-year-old man who had similar lesions removed one year before and returned with further papillomata. The specimen comprised several polyps, the largest (4 × 2 cm) with oedematous stroma and opaque thick surface epithelium of both transitional-cell and squamous-cell types.

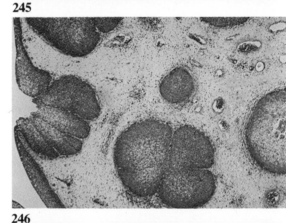

245 Antrochoanal 'inverted' papilloma (8120) One of several polyps removed at the time of submucous resection of the nasal septum from a 54-year-old fisherman. Section shows vascular chronic inflamed stroma with bulbous downgrowths of transitional epithelium. *(H&E × 13)*

246 Angiofibroma of the nasopharynx and antrum (9160) in a 19-year-old man, admitted with epistaxis. An irregularly lobulated firm mass (7 × 5.5 × 4.5 cm) with white to pale-brown cut surface showing darker brownish areas and an occasional cyst. Histologically it showed oedematous fibrous stroma containing stellate fibroblasts and numerous vascular channels, some with perivascular chronic inflammatory cell infiltrate, and appearances of juvenile angiofibroma.

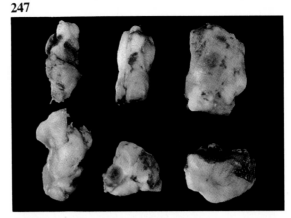

247 Plasmacytoma of the nose (9731) from a 59-year-old man who had nasal polyps which appeared rather dark in colour, solid and friable in parts. The specimen consists of six pieces, the largest being 2 cm long. Histologically these appeared to be made up entirely of plasma cells, some binucleate, others multinucleate and with mitotic activity, including abnormal forms. The surface epithelium was of upper respiratory type. The lesion was reported as plasmacytoma. Clinically it appeared to be an isolated lesion.

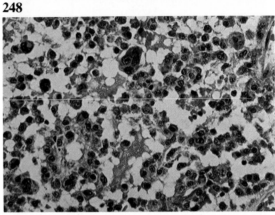

248 Plasmacytoma of the nasopharynx (9731) from an 84-year-old man who also had haemangiomas on his lip and tongue. He had mentioned the plum-coloured swelling in the back of his throat to his doctor 20 years ago but was advised to have nothing done: recently it had bled and the otolaryngologist removed it. The specimen was a (2 × 1.5 cm) soft mass with a smooth surface except at one pole where it was roughened. Section shows masses of plasma cells, some of near normal appearance, but many quite abnormal with two or more hyperchromatic nuclei. *(H&E × 133)*

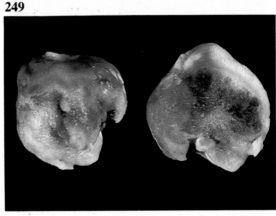

Larynx (T24)

249 Laryngeal nodule (Singer's node) (7381) from the right vocal cord of a 39-year-old man who complained of progressive hoarseness for four months. Micro-laryngoscopic excision of a large (16 × 16 × 12 mm) pedunculated polyp arising from the anterior third of the right vocal cord was carried out.

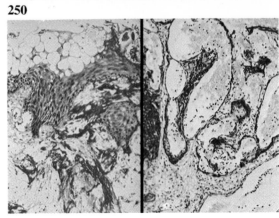

250 Laryngeal nodule (7381) Same lesion as shown in **249.** Section on left shows hydropic surface stratified squamous epithelium covering oedematous vascular stroma containing fibrinous deposits: on the right dilated vessels show fibrin (stained red) in their walls. *(H&E × 33) (MSB × 33)*

251

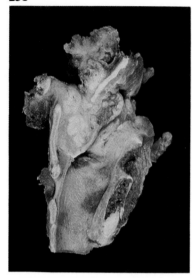

252

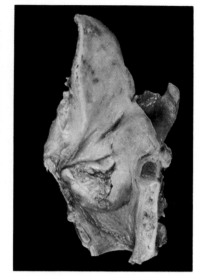

253

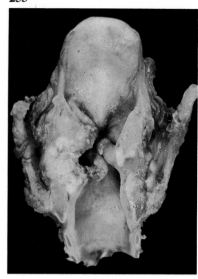

251 Supraglottic squamous-cell carcinoma (8073) of the larynx from a 62-year-old lorry driver, who had a squamous-cell carcinoma of the bronchus removed some months earlier. The specimen was a complete larynx including epiglottis, and included an ulcerated neoplasm which involved the posterior aspect of the epiglottis over an area (3.5 × 2 cm) extending from the right border across midline from near the apex downwards and posteriorly towards the arytenoid, leaving 10 to 15 mm of unaffected mucosa proximally and laterally. The rest of the mucosa of larynx and trachea appeared smooth. One parathyroid gland was identified on the posterior surface of the left lobe of the thyroid. Sections showed highly cellular (mitosis up to 20 per HP field) infiltrating squamous-cell carcinoma.

252 Squamous-cell carcinoma (8073) of the right vocal cord from a 69-year-old man who suffered hoarseness for six months and was treated by total laryngectomy. The specimen was received in two pieces: the right vocal cord was almost wholly destroyed by an ulcerated squamous-cell carcinoma (17 × 16 mm) infiltrating deeply, extending downwards to within 2.5 cm of the plane of resection.

253 Squamous-cell carcinoma (8073) of the vocal cords from a 65-year-old dock labourer who suffered hoarseness for six months. The specimen consists of complete larynx with epiglottis, two tracheal rings and hyoid bone. The left cord is ulcerated along its whole length and the anterior half of the right cord is roughened. The carcinoma (cryostat section showed squamous-cell carcinoma) excavates the pyriform fossa and marked vallecular oedema is present.

254

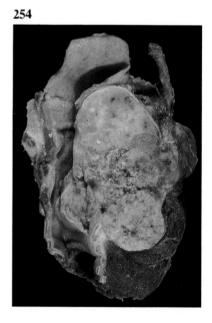

254 Chondrosarcoma of the larynx (9223) from a 73-year-old man who first complained of a swelling in his neck four years earlier. He became increasingly dyspnoeic and at laryngectomy a large (7 × 5 cm) bosselated cartilaginous tumour appeared to arise in the right thyroid cartilage, protruding into the larynx and narrowing the lumen to a 2 mm slit. It had a bluish-white cut surface and lobules of neoplasm infiltrated mucosa and adjacent muscles: some parts were gritty, yellowish and contained spicules of bone. Sections showed appearances of a low-grade chondrosarcoma, there being few mitoses but some cells with bizarre giant nuclei.

Lung (T28)

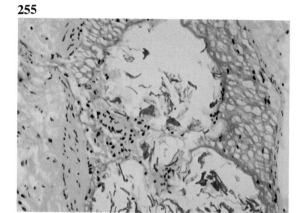

255   Amniotic fluid embolism (3714) Section of a lung from a woman who died shortly after delivery, in a state of hypofibrinogenaemia. Section is stained with Alcian phloxine to demonstrate mucin (green) and squames (red) derived from amniotic fluid in the pulmonary artery. Pulmonary oedema with collapse of both lungs was present. *(Alcian blue H. phlox T. ×83)*

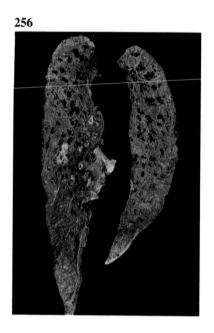

256   Pulmonary tuberculosis (4470) in a 64-year-old man believed to have carcinoma of left upper lobe and on whom thoracotomy and left upper lobectomy were carried out. The specimen is a left upper lobe of lung (weight 170g) with all but the lingular segment collapsed. A 2 cm diameter mass was palpable adjacent to the bronchus to the anterior segment and smaller nodules were present in the subapical region. The specimen was fixed by infusing with formalin and sliced exposing a tuberculoma. There was focal anthracotic scarring and emphysema and small caseous foci. AAFB were present (up to 30 per HP field) in caseous exudate in the lumen of the tertiary bronchus on which the tuberculoma encroached. The lesions were fibro-caseous with peripheral activity as evidenced by tuber-culoid granulomata with Langhans' giant cells extending along alveolar walls and into peribronchial tissues. *No* carcinoma was found.

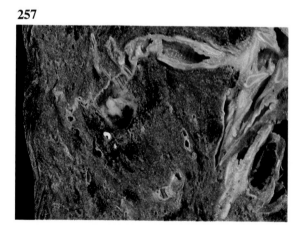

257   Tuberculoma (4470) Close-up of the same lesion as in **256** at a deeper level. The caseous lesion encroaches on the tertiary bronchus. The dense white areas are caused by calcification.

258

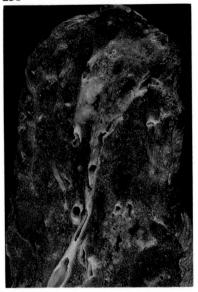

259

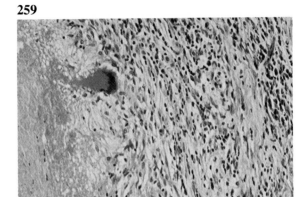

259 Pulmonary tuberculosis (4470) A section from the lesion in **258** shows caseating lesion with Langhans' giant cell, epithelioid cells, lymphocytes and plasma cells and fibrous tissue with few blood vessels. *(H&E × 53)*

258 Pulmonary tuberculosis (4470) in a 45-year-old woman believed to have carcinoma of right upper lobe and on whom thoracotomy and right upper lobectomy were performed. The specimen was fixed by instillation of formalin then sliced, exposing multiple calcified caseous foci with well-developed fibrous capsule; but in the upper segment, 2cm from the upper border, a pale greyish-pink area 15 × 9mm shows small satellite nodules. Histological section shows evidence of active pulmonary tuberculosis with recent follicular lesions in the wall of alveoli and bronchial mucosa and scanty AAFB. Sections of a lymph node showed follicular tuberculoid granulomas. *No* carcinoma was found.

260

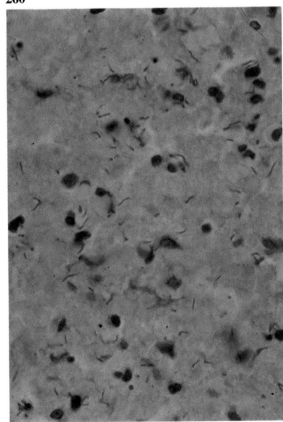

260 Pulmonary tuberculosis (4470) A section of caseous exudate from a bronchus stained by Ziehl-Neelsen's method. There are numerous acid alcohol fast bacilli (AAFB) morphologically indistinguishable from Mycobacterium tuberculosis. *(Ziehl-Neelsen × 330)*

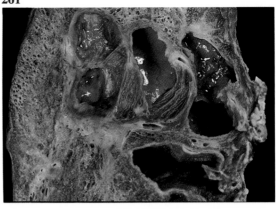

261 Aspergillus mycetoma (E 4323) **with bronchiectasis** (3412) from a woman with a suspicious lesion in the left upper lobe. Left lower lobectomy was done and the bronchus to the apical/subapical segment exuded dark-brown to green sticky fluid, which on culture grew an Aspergillus. After fixation the specimen was sliced, exposing *no* neoplasm but severe bronchiectasis (dilatation up to 9mm), some of the cavities being filled with brown mycetoma. Histologically granulomatous lesions were present in the chronically inflamed walls of the ectatic bronchi. No AAFB were identified.

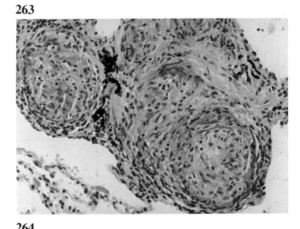

262 Aspergillus (E 4323) fruiting head and spores from a pneumonic area in a patient dying with aspergillus pneumonia. *(Gomori methenamine silver × 330)*

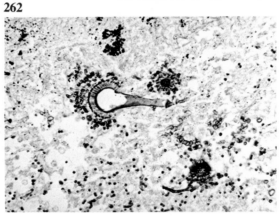

263 Sarcoidosis (4454) Needle biopsy from a 55-year-old woman with bilateral pulmonary infiltrate on xray, and suffering from rheumatoid arthritis. The sections showed no evidence of rheumatoid lung but there were multiple non-caseating follicular granulomas in which lymphocytes were scanty and no AAFB were demonstrated in Ziehl-Neelsen-stained sections. *(H&E × 83)*

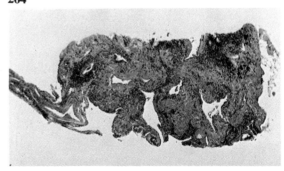

264 Fibrosing alveolitis (4815) Needle biopsy from 68-year-old man with history of treatment for pulmonary tuberculosis when aged 38, and diagnosed as having fibrosing alveolitis when aged 53. Recent respiratory distress led to cytological examination of sputum and a report of query alveolar carcinoma. Bronchoscopy proved negative, a needle biopsy showed marked thickening of alveolar walls, non-specific chronic inflammation and fibrosis. *No* carcinoma was seen. *(H&E × 13)*

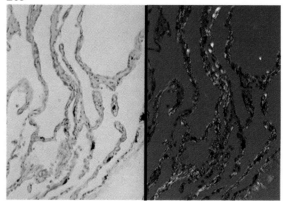

265 Amyloidosis of lung (5515) Section stained with congo red viewed on left with ordinary light and on right with polarising microscope shows dichroic birefringence. The patient had suffered from Crohn's disease for over 20 years and had very extensive secondary amyloidosis. *(Congo red ×53)*

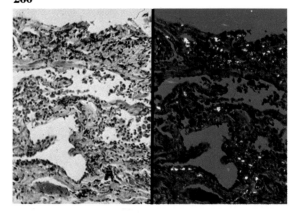

266 Anthracosilicosis of lung (5604) A section of needle biopsy from a case of silicosis. The silica particles are birefringent and stand out very conspicuously when viewed (right) with partial polarised light. *(H&E×53)*

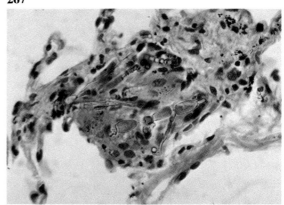

267 Asbestosis of lung (5611) A section of needle biopsy from a case of asbestosis. The fibres become coated with iron-containing protein to form the characteristic segmented golden-yellow bodies shown here. *(H&E×133)*

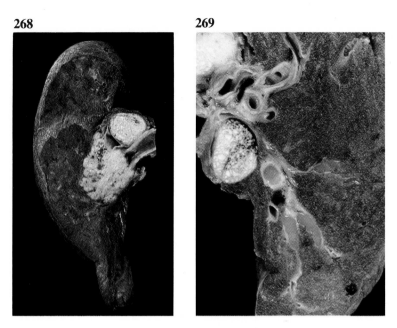

268

269

268 Bronchial carcinoma (8073) from a 68-year-old man with a 4 cm tumour involving the distal part of the left main-stem bronchus growing into and blocking the lumen of the bronchus to the posterior basic segment. Enlarged nodes (5 and 3.5 cm) at the hilum appeared replaced by metastases. The sections showed highly cellular (mitoses up to 30 per HP field) anaplastic squamous-cell carcinoma with occasional areas showing glandular differentiation. Basophilic masses of nucleic acid were present in areas of necrosis.

269 Bronchial carcinoma (8073) Deeper plane of section of same specimen as **268** to show enlarged hilar node replaced by metastases and bronchiectasis distal to it.

270

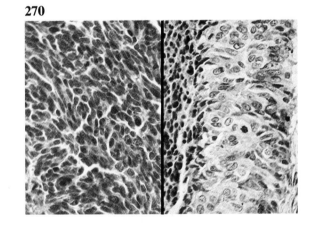

270 Bronchial carcinoma (8043) (8073) Sections showing on left 'oat-cell' type of carcinoma, on right anaplastic squamous-cell carcinoma. *(H&E × 133)*

271

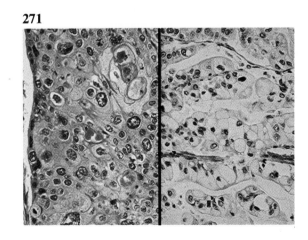

271 Carcinoma of lung (8073) (8143) Sections showing on the left moderately well-differentiated squamous-cell carcinoma, and on the right adenocarcinoma. *(H&E × 113)*

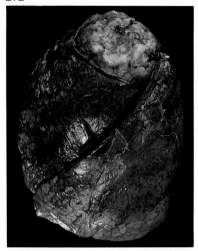

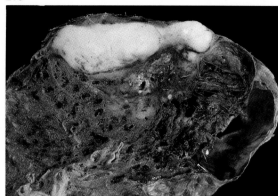

273 Carcinoma of lung (8143) Close up of the cut surface of the lesion in **272** showing close relationship of the (9 × 3 cm) carcinoma to the pigmented scar and also the bullous emphysema.

272 Carcinoma of lung (8143) from a 58-year-old man with Pancoast's syndrome. The left pneumonectomy specimen showed a 9 cm neoplastic plaque at the apex and there were large (6 cm) emphysematous bullae along the anterior border of the upper lobe and string-like interlobar adhesions. The cut surface showed widespread emphysema, pigmentation and scarring and the neoplasm appears to arise in relation to a scar

(2 × 1.3 cm) at the apex. Histologically the lesion was reported as a poorly differentiated glandular carcinoma. The cut end of bronchus appeared free of neoplasm.

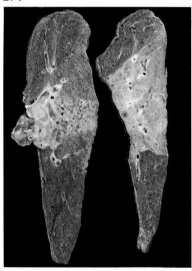

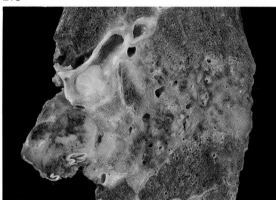

275 Bronchial carcinoid (8240) Close up of the same lesion in **274** showing yellow tumour, lipid pneumonia and reactive enlarged nodes.

274 Bronchial carcinoid tumour (8240) from a 34-year-old woman heavy cigarette smoker. A right upper lobectomy was done. The specimen weighs 215 g, measures 16 × 12 × 6 cm, and shows enlarged black and grey nodes at the hilum. The middle third of the specimen, corresponding to the anterior segment, is consolidated and partly collapsed, the pleura showing a red-to-yellow granularity. A slice through the main bronchus to upper lobe reveals a near spherical mass (9 mm in diameter) bulging into the lumen, from

between cartilages and with its base (within 3 mm of the plane of excision) astride the bifurcation of the first division bronchus to the anterior segment. The cut surface has a yellow nodular appearance. The lung shows typical changes of lipid pneumonia confirmed on frozen section. Histologically the bronchial lesion shows appearance of a bronchial carcinoid tumour. *No* metastases were seen in sections of the enlarged nodes. There was *no* excess 5H1AA in the urine.

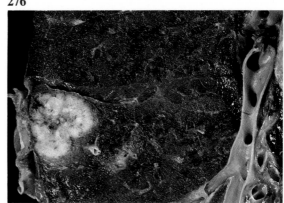

276 Carcinoma of lung (8483) from a man with a peripherally placed 'coin' lesion. The pneumonectomy specimen showed neoplastic tissue on the pleural surface of the posterolateral aspect of the apical segment of the lower lobe, overlying the primary carcinoma (2.3 cm) which histologically was a mucin producing adenocarcinoma. Metastases in pleural lymphatics and in hilar nodes were present. The possibility of the lesion being metastatic could not be excluded, though no alimentary lesion was apparent.

277

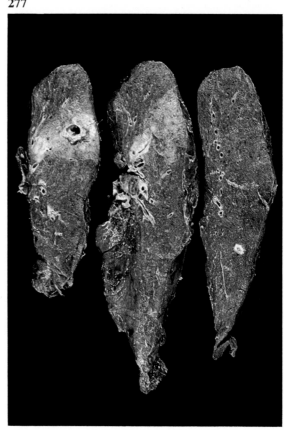

277 Carcinoma of lung (8563) from a 43-year-old woman who complained of weight loss and malaise, with radio-opacities in the left upper lobe. Sputum contained malignant cells suggestive of adenocarcinoma. The left upper-lobectomy specimen shows a cavity surrounded by pale neoplasm in an area supplied by the subapical segmental bronchus, which shows circumferential involvement by pale solid neoplasm beginning 2 cm from the plane of resection. One hilar node contained metastases and in one slice a solitary small (9 × 6 mm) metastasis is seen situated 1.3 cm beneath the pleura 5 cm from the hilum in the lower part of the specimen. Histologically the carcinoma showed an extraordinary variation in pattern, ranging from epidermoid through transitional to columnar cell glandular with undifferentiated areas as well. The discrete metastasis showed glandular differentiation.

4 Cardiovascular system

Artery (T41)

278 Post-irradiation damage (1130) to an ovarian artery from a 27-year-old woman treated for cervical carcinoma with radiotherapy three weeks before hysterectomy. Section shows recanalised thrombus with much haemosiderin and bizarre large histiocytes with dense darkly staining nuclei. *(H&E × 53)*

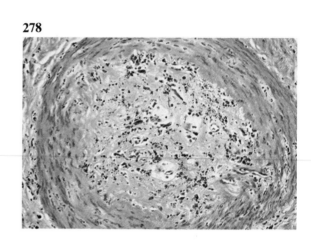

278

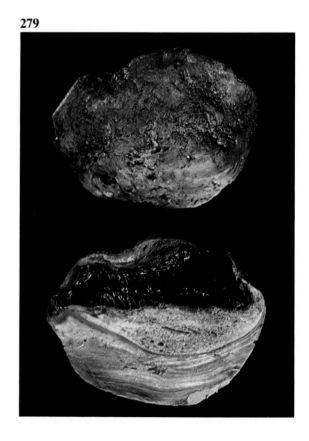

279

279 Laminated thrombus (3702) excised from an aortic aneurysm from a 78-year-old man and showing typical laminated structure with striae – the lines of Zahn. It measured 12 × 9 cm and the lumen at one end was approximately 7 cm wide narrowing to 2 cm at the other.

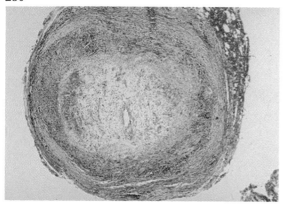

280 Giant-cell arteritis (temporal arteritis) (4922)
Section to show circumferential inflammation with
focal medial necrosis, giant-cell reaction, organising
thrombus in the intima and narrowed lumen.
(H&E × 13)

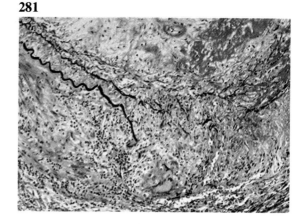

281 Giant-cell arteritis (temporal arteritis) (4922)
Section to show segment of same artery as in **280** with
breaks in elastic lamina and multinucleate giant cell
applied to free end of an elastic lamina. The media
shows an area of necrosis (loss of nuclear staining) and
there is fibrin insudation in media and intima. *(Elastica
H&E × 53)*

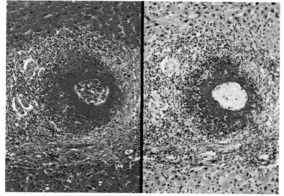

282 Polyarteritis nodosa (4924) Sections to show
changes in hepatic artery from same case as in **283**.
(H&E on left, MSB on right × 33)

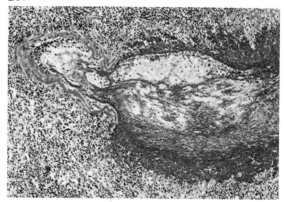

283 Polyarteritis nodosa (4924) Section to show
exudation of fibrin (stained red) through affected
segment of renal artery wall. *(MSB × 13)*

284 Periarteritis nodosa (4924) A section of biopsy of
a deltoid muscle from a 36-year-old man who suffered
disabling rheumatoid arthritis for nine years, was on
steroids and also severely hypertensive. Section shows
a small (150 micron diameter) artery with dense focal
leucocytic (monocytes, lymphocytes, occasional plasma
cell and eosinophil polymorphonuclear) infiltration
especially of the adventitia and media: neutrophil
polymorphonuclear leucocytes were scanty, more
obvious towards the intima. *(H&E × 53)*

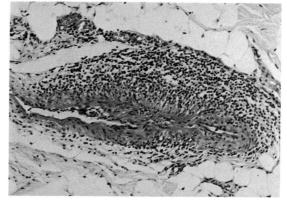

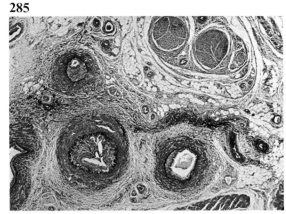

285

285 Buerger's disease (thromboangiitis obliterans) (4537) Section of a neurovascular bundle from an amputated leg. The section shows artery with intact elastic lamina and recanalised lumen: both venae comitantes show intimal thickening and the nerve shows perineurial and epineurial thickening. *(Elastica H&E × 6)*

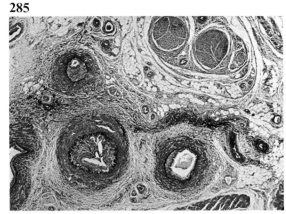

286

286 Buerger's disease (4537) Section of an artery from the same specimen as in **285**. Section shows part of an artery with heavy inflammatory cell infiltration of the wall. In some areas multinucleate macrophages were present. *(Elastica H&E × 53)*

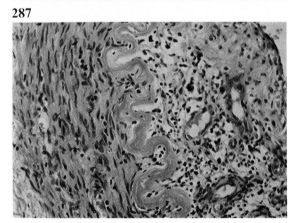

287

287 Buerger's disease (4537) Section of an artery from the same specimen as in **285**. Section shows new vessel formation in wall (media and intima) and mononuclear cell inflammatory infiltrate (lymphocytes and plasma cells). The elastic lamina is thickened but intact. *(H&E × 83)*

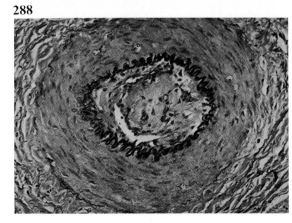

288

288 Buerger's disease (4537) Section of a digital artery showing almost complete occlusion by organising thrombus: it is unusual to see such appearances in digital arteries from cases with limb ischaemia caused by atheroma. *(Elastica H&E × 83)*

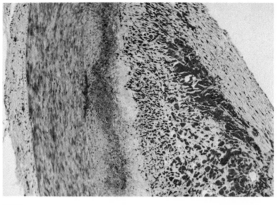

289   Atheroma (5212) Frozen section of atheromatous artery to show accumulation of lipid in the intima. It shows fibrous layer over the fatty plaque in which intracellular and extracellular lipids are seen; there appears to be some 'hold up' of lipid along one short length of the internal elastic lamina. *(Oil red O haemalum ×53)*

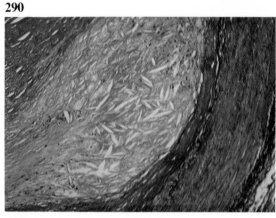

290   Atheroma (5212) Paraffin section of atheromatous artery to show sterol clefts in atheromatous plaque in the intima in a section of a paraffin-processed block. *(Elastica H&E ×53)*

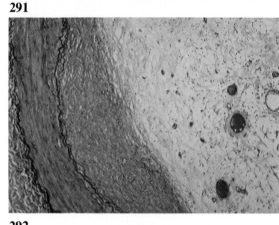

291   Atheroma (5212) Section of recanalised atheromatous artery, showing thin-walled vessels in loose fibroblastic tissue, which is separated from internal elastic lamina by fairly cellular tissue including fibrocytic and smooth muscle cells. *(Elastica H&E ×53)*

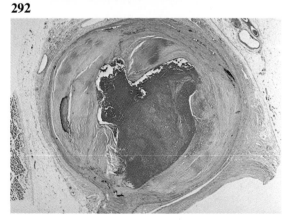

292   Atheroma with recent thrombo-occlusion (5212) Section shows circumferential thickening of intima, patchy calcification of the plaques and marked atrophy of media, of this femoral artery from a patient with gangrene of leg and foot. The lumen is filled with recent thrombus in which (bottom centre) atheromatous debris, including sterol clefts, is present. *(H&E ×3)*

293

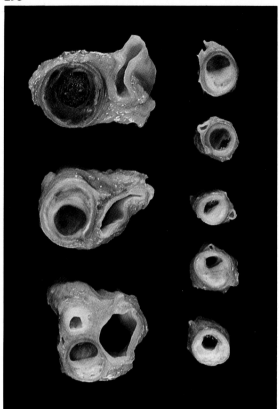

293   Atheroma and thromboembolism (5212) in the artery of a lower limb from an old man with myocardial infarct and mural thrombus. The sections show recent red thromboembolus in the femoral artery (the largest vessel top left) and atheroma of varying age and colour in the distal arteries. Some plaques are brown or yellow, others are white and the cut surface shows the characteristic signet-ring appearance.

294

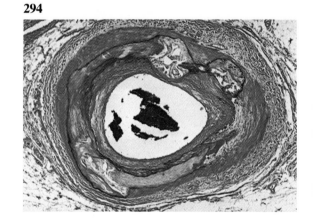

294   Medial calcification of dorsalis pedis artery (5242) from an amputated gangrenous foot. Section shows extensive medial calcification but the lumen is still quite patent. The cause of the gangrene was femoral and popliteal artery thrombosis complicating severe atheroma. *(H&E × 13)*

5   Digestive glands

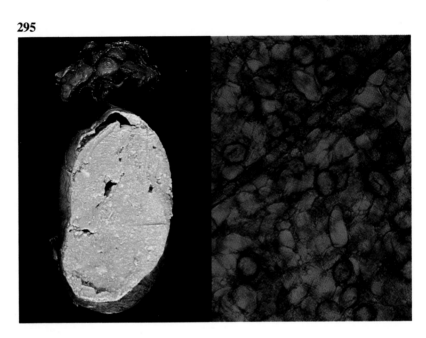

295

Mouth (T51)

295   Dermoid cyst (9080) from the floor of the mouth of a trainee nurse. The cyst had become larger and when excised measured 6×3 cm; the contents were yellow-cheesy material with a few hairs arising from pilosebaceous follicles in the wall. On the right contents viewed with polarising light and first order red compensator show keratinised squamous and a hair shaft. (×53)

296

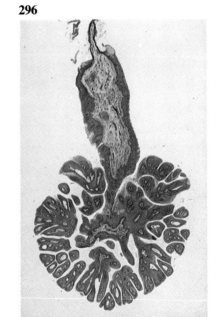

296   Squamous papilloma (8070) of the uvula from a 36-year-old woman. Section shows the almost spherical (4 mm) lesion on a narrow (4 mm) pedicle. (H&E × 3.5)

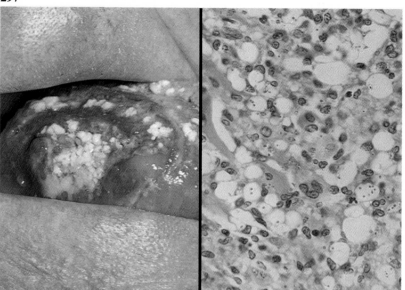

Tongue (T53)

297 Histoplasmosis of tongue (4400) in a 71-year-old retired jute worker who complained of painful ulceration of the tongue for four months. Despite a biopsy diagnosis of a fungal granulomatous lesion, the patient's general surgeon opted to do a hemi-glossectomy. The following day the patient died in adrenal failure (the adrenals were grossly affected by histoplasmosis as were the lungs). The section shows the capsulate yeast-like forms of Histoplasma lying free and in macrophages in tissue from the base of the (4 × 3 cm) ulcer. *(H&E × 83)*

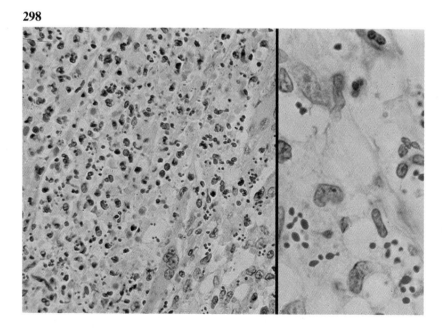

298 Histoplasmosis of tongue (4400) Section of an ulcer stained by 'Red Gram' method in which the Gram-positive Histoplasma appear as bright red yeast-like ovoid bodies: budding forms are shown on the right. *('Red Gram' × 53 × 330)*

299 **Rhomboid median chronic glossitis** (7324) Lesion excised from a 52-year-old man who was worried about an 'ulcer in the middle at the back of his tongue'. Clinically the lesion was not ulcerated and histologically there was acanthosis and non-specific chronic inflammation without demonstrable fungi or other microorganisms. *(H&E × 13)*

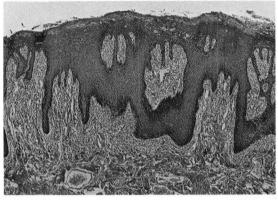

300

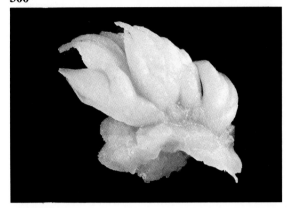

300 **Squamous-cell papilloma** (8070) of the tongue from a 73-year-old woman who had been aware of the white projection on top of her tongue for several years. The (7 × 4 mm) lesion was histologically a simple keratinising squamous-cell papilloma. *(× 3.5)*

301

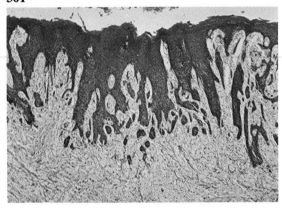

301 **Granular-cell myoblastoma of the tongue** (9370) Section shows characteristic pseudoepitheliomatous hyperplasia of the squamous epithelium overlying the tumour. *(H&E × 13)*

302

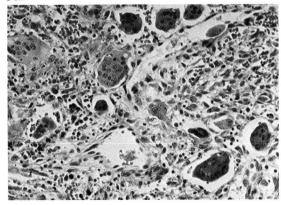

Gingiva (T54)

302 **Myeloid epulis** (7386) from the gingiva of a young girl. Section shows multinucleate giant cells (?odontoblasts) spindle cells, haemosiderophages and recent haemorrhage. The child was not on any drugs and there was no detectable upset in dentition or calcium and phosphorus metabolism. Excision was curative. *(H&E × 83)*

Salivary gland (T55)

303 Chronic sialadenitis with calculus (4300) from submandibular gland. Sialograms showed presence of obstruction by calculus. The specimen shows the (4.5 × 3 × 2 cm) gland with cream-coloured 2 × 1.4 cm calculus tightly wedged in the salivary duct, which histologically showed squamous metaplasia. There were low-grade chronic inflammatory changes throughout the gland.

304 Adenolymphoma (Warthin's tumour) (8560) from the angle of the jaw of a 73-year-old man, who gave a history that the lump had slowly increased in size during the last nine months. Blood film had shown a lymphocytosis and a clinical diagnosis of tuberculous cervical adenitis was made. The specimen is a mass (5.5 × 3 × 2 cm) with smooth surface. On gross section the surface appears loculated with paler whitish bands surrounding clefts and wider spaces filled with light pinkish-brown homogeneous material. Sections confirmed the pathologist's naked-eye diagnosis of adenolymphoma.

305 Adenolymphoma (Warthin's tumour) (8560) Section of another example showing the typical combination of epithelial and lymphoid elements, with clefts containing secretion. A small piece of salivary gland (arrowed) can be seen at bottom left of the section. *(H&E × 2)*

306 Adenolymphoma (Warthin's tumour) (8560) from a 61-year-old female. Section shows (top left) part of a germinal centre, then a cuff of lymphocytes with two duct-like structures containing double-layered tall epithelial cells with pale staining cytoplasm. However, several of the tall cells show dense eosinophilia of their cytoplasm and the nuclei appear small and darkly stained. *(H&E × 83)*

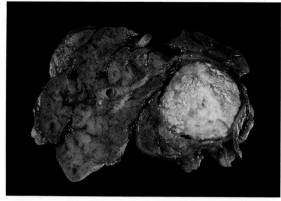
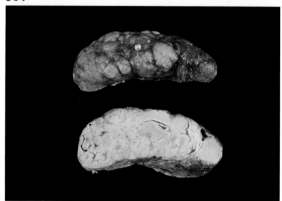
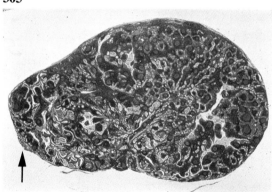
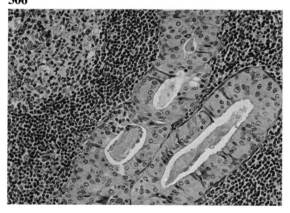

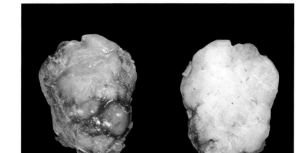

307 Pleomorphic salivary adenoma (mixed parotid tumour) (8940) from a 35-year-old woman with a history of a slowly increasing painless swelling in the region of the parotid gland. The specimen is a (3.5×2.5×2 cm) lobulated mass with bluish-white glistening cut surface; in places it looks quite like cartilage.

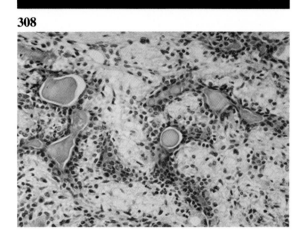

308 Pleomorphic salivary adenoma (8940) Section of the lesion shown in **307** shows various types of epithelium forming irregular patterns and stroma appearing loose and myxomatous – in other areas it was more fibrous and collagenous; chondroid differentiation and calcification were also noted. Mitoses were scanty and no evidence of malignancy was seen. *(H&E ×53)*

Liver (T56)

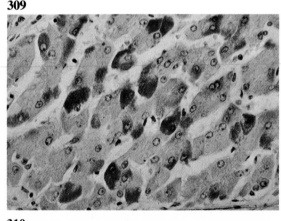

309 Viral hepatitis (E 3918) Section stained with orcein (normally used as a stain for elastic tissue) which stains affected liver cells a dark brown colour. In H&E sections 'ground glass change' is seen, the cell cytoplasm appearing more or less eosinophilic and finely granular and with dislocated nucleus. Orcein-positive ground glass change is so far only described in HBs Ag positive patients. *(Mod. orcein ×83)*

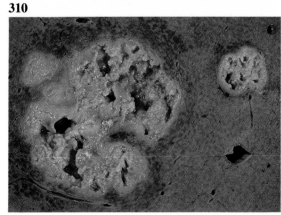

310 Amoebic hepatitis (4174) with multiple abscesses 1–3 cm from same case as in **13**. The contents of the abscess are usually described as resembling anchovy sauce. Amoebae can usually be demonstrated in the hepatic parenchyma around such abscesses.

311 Hepatic cirrhosis and porphyria cutanea tarda
(4850) Liver biopsy taken during an episode of
cholestatic jaundice probably caused by chlorproma-
zine. The diagnosis of porphyria had been established
six years earlier when unstained cryostat section of liver
biopsy showed red fluorescence when viewed with blue
light (400 nm). *(× 180)*

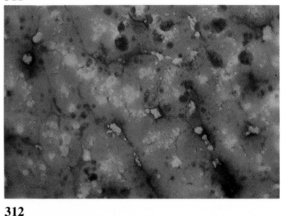

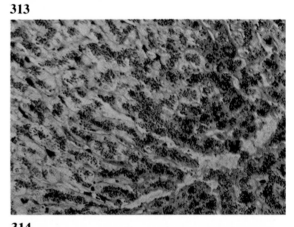

312 Wilson's disease (5053) Liver sections from a
child with hepatolenticular degeneration. On the left
stained with DMABR which gives a distinct brick red
colour with copper containing granules. *(p-dimethyl-
amino benzylidine rhodanine × 133)*

On the right stained with Timm's silver sulphide
technique which produces brown-to-black colour with
copper. This technique is easily the most sensitive for
demonstrating copper in tissue sections. *(Timm's × 133)*

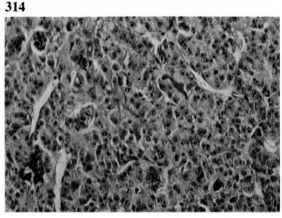

313 Haemochromatosis (bronze diabetes) (5741)
Section of liver showing haemosiderin granules in
parenchymal cells, in connective tissues (there is always
cirrhosis) in Kupffer cells and other phagocytic cells.
Staining with Perls' stain shows a positive prussian blue
reaction at these sites. *(Perls' scarba red × 83)*

314 Hepatocarcinoma (8173) Section to show green
bile accumulation in canaliculi and ductules formed
between columns of neoplastic cells. *(van Gieson × 83)*

315 **Hepatocarcinoma (malignant hepatoma)** (8173) from a 66-year-old man. An extended hemihepatectomy specimen weighing 1525g and measuring 26 × 18 × 10cm has a roughly spherical circumscribed tumour just deep to the capsule in the right lobe. A rim of non-neoplastic hepatic tissue is present all round. Histologically it was reported as a well-differentiated hepatocellular carcinoma, in places almost indistinguishable from normal, elsewhere it showed acinar arrangement or unorganised masses of polyhedral cells. The neoplasm appeared free of haemosiderin but the hepatic parenchymal cells

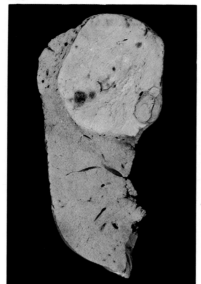

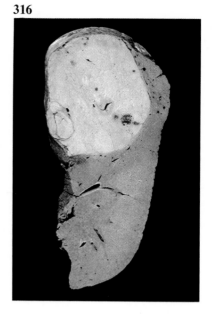

contained moderate quantities but not enough for a diagnosis of haemochromatosis. This patient, like many others with iron-storage problems, worked in a licensed premises.

316 **Hepatocarcinoma** (8173) Same specimen as shown in **315** stained with Perls' reagent to demonstrate hepatic siderosis, while the neoplasm appears more or less free of haemosiderin.

317 **Hepatoblastoma** (8973) from a two-year-old boy with progressive anaemia, tiredness and large mass in right hypochondrium. Partial hepatectomy was carried out. The specimen weighed 1160g, measured 17 × 15 × 10cm and most of its bulk was made up of two neoplastic masses (each about 10cm in diameter). One to the right is friable with dark red, brown and yellowish variegated cut surface, the other to the left is firmer and nodular with greenish tinge. Histologically the appearances were reported as those of hepatoblastoma with some areas of well-differentiated polyhedral cells resembling normal hepatocytes, but others showing quite undifferentiated proliferating malignant cells. The boy died 18 months later with pulmonary metastases.

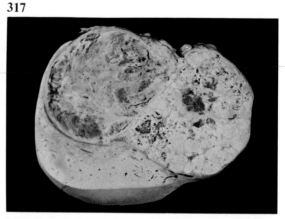

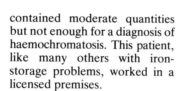

318 **Hepatoblastoma** (8973) Section of a specimen from the lesion shown in **317** to show appearance in the well-differentiated areas where the neoplasm consists of polyhedral cells arranged in trabeculae and lobules. *(H&E × 83)*

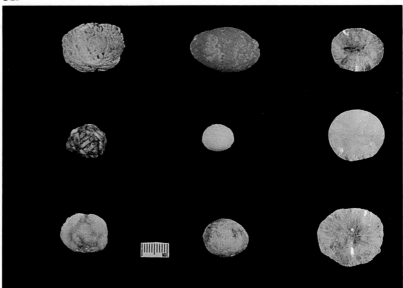

Gallbladder (T57)

319   Gallstones (3102) A selection of 'solitary pure sterol' gallstones. They are from 1 to 3 cm long, usually ovoid and transparent: the surface is either smooth or beset with crystal blocks, sometimes yellowish due to small amounts of incorporated bile pigment. They usually show radial striation.

320

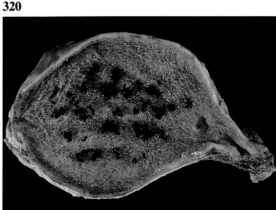

320   Gallstones (3104) Calcium bilirubinate gallstones in the mildly inflamed gallbladder from a 46-year-old man. These are in the form of thin brittle twiglike branches up to 8 mm long.

321

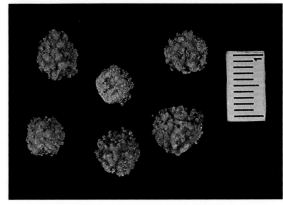

321   Gallstones (3101) Calcium carbonate gallstones. These small (5 mm) very hard mulberry like stones were removed from a shrunken chronically inflamed gallbladder. They are mainly calcium carbonate with some cholesterol.

322

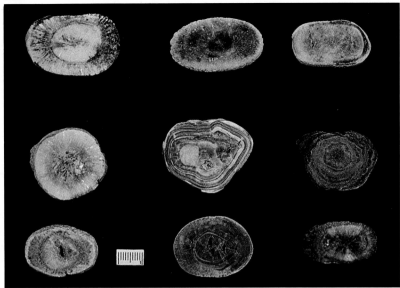

322 Gallstones (3106) A selection of 'solitary' mixed gallstones. They are from 3 to 5 cm long, usually ovoid and opaque. The surface is usually smooth or finely granular. Sterol predominates but laminae rich in pigment are common. They look quite like agate on cross-section.

323

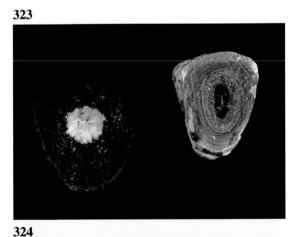

323 Gallstones (3106) On the left a composite gallstone 18 mm in diameter with a 'pure sterol' core and 'pure pigment' shell. On the right a composite gallstone from a patient who suffered from non-spherocytic haemolytic anaemia and produced the gallstones as evidence! The pigment core would certainly corroborate a story of some haemolytic episode in the past.

324

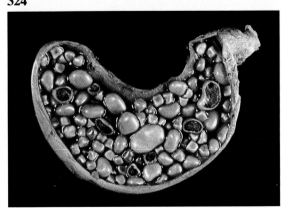

324 Chronic cholecystitis (3106) with mixed sterol and pigment gallstones from a 66-year-old woman who complained of epigastric pain, nausea, vomiting and diarrhoea; multiple gallstones were seen on xray. The thin-walled gallbladder is 8 cm long, up to 3 cm in diameter and is filled with green bile and 200 pearly gallstones of mixed sterol and pigment type.

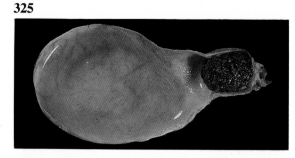

325 Mucocoele of gallbladder (3526) with solitary stone (2 × 1.4 cm) impacted in Hartman's pouch.

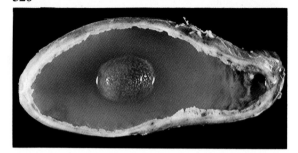

326 Chronic cholecystitis (3526) with solitary sterol stone (2.5 × 1.5 cm) floating in clear mucoid bile. The wall is thickened and obviously inflamed with areas of congestion, haemorrhage, mural oedema, dilated Rokitansky-Aschoff sinuses and mucosal ulceration.

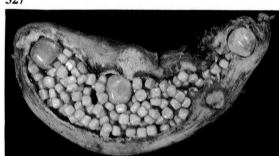

327 Empyema of the gallbladder (4045), with perforation, from a 76-year-old woman who complained of hypochondrial pain and with a palpable gallbladder full of pus and facetted gallstones of mixed sterol and pigment type, many of them the size and shape of corn grains; others were larger, up to 1.5 cm in diameter. The thickened wall (1.2 cm) shows several abscess cavities, from which coliform organisms were cultured.

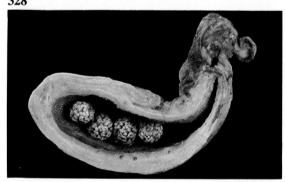

328 Chronic cholecystitis (4300) with multiple mulberry yellow-grey gallstones (mainly sterol), up to 8 mm in diameter. The wall is thick (up to 8 mm) and there are cysts in the wall, both in the body and at the fundus. Histologically there was severe chronic cholecystitis, and inflammation around Rokitansky-Aschoff sinuses.

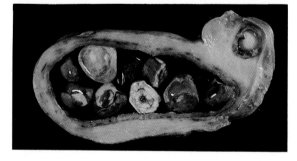

329 Chronic cholecystitis (4300) with multiple mixed (sterol and pigment) gallstones, from 0.7 to 1.7 cm in diameter. The gallbladder, 11 cm long with thick wall (up to 1 cm) due to oedema, fibrosis and chronic inflammation was non-functioning; its removal cured the 64-year-old woman's pain in the right upper abdomen.

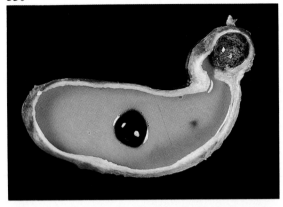

330   Chronic cholecystitis (4400) with multiple facetted gallstones of mixed type, pigment and sterol, from 6 mm to 20 mm diameter. The bile looked like mustard and the wall appeared very pale and thickened. One stone is impacted in the cystic duct. The sections showed granulomatous foci around sterol crystals in the wall.

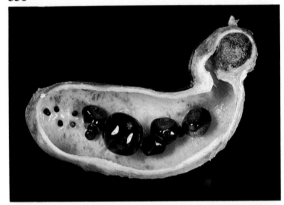

331   Chronic cholecystitis (4400) Same specimen as in 330 after draining away the contents which were sterile on culture and showed abundant sterol crystals without purulent exudate. Infective empyema of the gallbladder is quite uncommon.

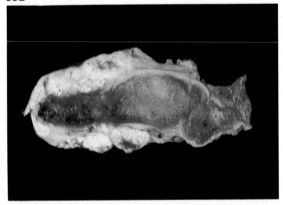

332   Xanthogranulomatous cholecystitis (4400) suspected as carcinoma because of the greatly thickened and indurated wall: cryostat section, however, showed that the appearances were caused by granuloma formation and accumulation of sterol-containing macrophages. No evidence of malignancy was found in many paraffin sections.

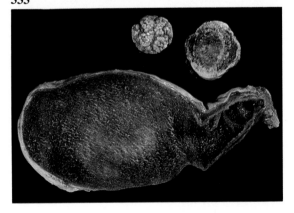

333   Cholesterolosis of gallbladder (5524) with two mixed sterol and pigment stones (2 cm and 1.4 cm in diameter).

334

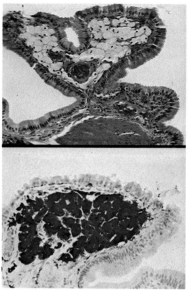

334 Cholesterolosis of gallbladder (5524) Section showing lipid-containing macrophages in the lamina propria: top shows H&E paraffin section – the cells appear clear because the lipid has been dissolved out in processing, bottom shows cryostat section stained with Oil red O. *(×53)*

335

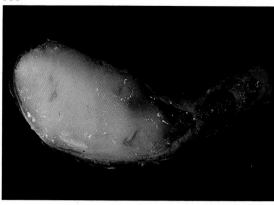

335 Lime-water bile in chronic cholecystitis (5541) from a 31-year-old woman with a two-year history of intermittent pain. Radiologist reported non-functioning gallbladder. An 11cm long gallbladder full of white lime-water bile and with a (2×1cm) solitary sterol stone impacted in the cystic duct. Calcification was present in the wall.

336 Cholecystitis with adenomyosis (7672) and facetted mixed pigment and sterol gallstones (up to 2.1cm) from a 64-year-old woman with a one-year history of pain in hypochondrium radiating to the back, and accompanying flatulent dyspepsia. The gallbladder is 11cm long with speckled red serosa. The contents are mucoid brown bile and three facetted gallstones. The wall is thickened (from 3 to 6mm) with many Rokitansky-Aschoff sinuses and cysts towards the fundus (so called adenomyosis).

336

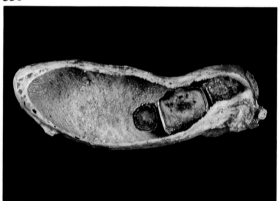

337

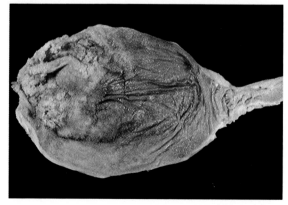

337 Carcinoma of the gallbladder (8143) from an 86-year-old woman who complained of colicky upper abdominal pain off and on for five years; there was tenderness to deep palpation in the right hypochondrium. She died suddenly before surgery could be attempted. At necropsy the gallbladder at the fundus was adherent to the liver, there being direct infiltration of the liver by adenocarcinoma of the gallbladder. There was some pigment gravel among the green-brown bile but no large stones. There were no metastases elsewhere. The cause of death was cerebral embolism from mitral valve infective endocarditis.

Pancreas (T59)

338 Chronic pancreatitis (4300) suspected as carcinoma. The specimen is a (10 × 4 cm) mass of pancreas weighing 180 g. The cut surface is white with creamy areas here and there where some pancreatic lobules have survived. Ducts were irregular in calibre, some of them dilated. Histologically *no* evidence of malignancy was found, there being loss of acinar tissue, fibrosis, and prominence of islets of Langerhans.

339 Carcinoma of the head of the pancreas (8653) in a 72-year-old man with obstructive jaundice: at operation a grossly dilated common bile duct and a large 3 cm carcinoma was found in the head of the pancreas and ulcerating through into the duodenum: the ampulla of Vater was intact 12 mm beyond the most distal part of the ulcerated neoplasm. Histologically it was a glandular carcinoma, but showed a varied pattern ranging from undifferentiated spheroidal cells to acini and tubules of columnar cells as well as areas of squamous-cell differentiation.

340 Pancreatic cystadenoma (8440) from an 89-year-old woman with a six-year history of a mass in the left hypochondrium. Recent loss of appetite had made the patient seek advice. Clinically it was thought to be a cystic carcinoma, but the bosselated cystic mass (15 × 11 × 9 cm) weighing 700 g with sponge-like cut surface proved on histological examination to be a benign cystadenoma: apparently normal islets were present in parts of the lesion.

338

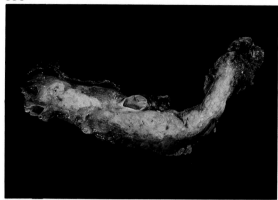

339

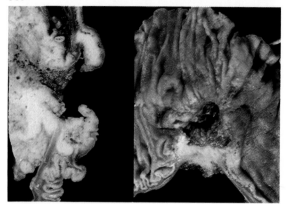

340

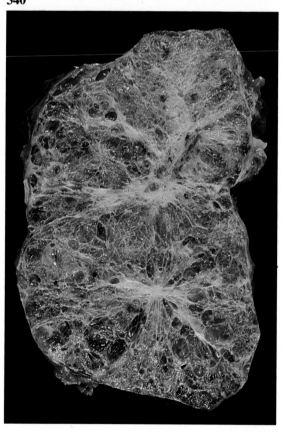

6 Gastrointestinal tract

Tonsil (T61)

341 Reticulum cell sarcoma (9643) of the tonsil
(diffuse histiocytic lymphoma) from a 55-year-old man
with a history of feeling a lump in his throat for 12
weeks. The tonsil was received in two pieces: the larger
piece was $5 \times 3 \times 2$ cm and the smaller piece was
$3.5 \times 2.5 \times 2$ cm. The cut surface was pale and homogeneous. Initial report was framed as undifferentiated
malignant neoplasm: after examining plastic embedded
sections and electronmicrographs, the general agreement was that this was a sarcoma.

342 Malignant neoplasm (8016) in supraclavicular
node ?sarcoma ?carcinoma. The woman complained of
a recent (two week) history of a painless swelling in the
neck. A biopsy of an enlarged node was reported as
malignant but of uncertain type. A repeat biopsy one
week later produced paraffin sections which again
failed to allow a definite diagnosis. Electronmicrographs
showed appearances which strongly favoured a
diagnosis of metastatic carcinoma (see **343**) from tonsil
or pharynx. *(H&E × 133)*

343 Metastatic carcinoma (8016) Same lesion as in
342. Electronmicrograph showing 3 desmosomes
(arrowed). *(× 25,000)*

341

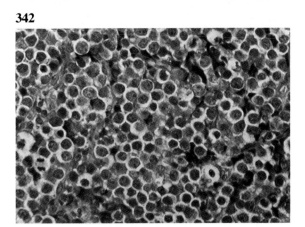

342

343

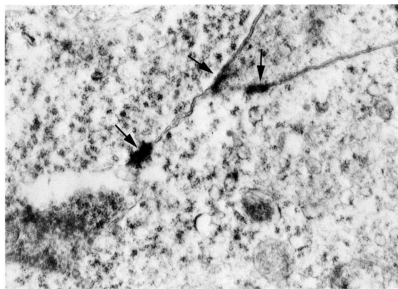

Oesophagus (T62)

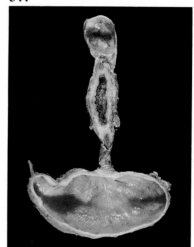

344 Duplication of oesophagus and stomach (2810) from a young boy with a webbed neck, and a history of anaemia from repeated gastrointestinal bleeding. Peptic ulceration was evident in the oesophageal duplication.

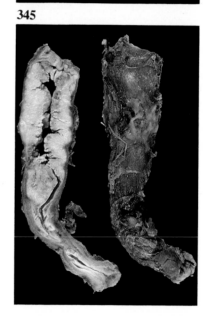

345 Carcinoma of oesophagus (8073) from a 69-year-old woman with severe dysphagia: radiologically a malignant stricture was demonstrated. The specimen consisted of middle third of oesophagus measuring, after fixation, 11 cm: 6.5 cm of the length of the segment is invaded by a squamous-cell carcinoma reaching to within 5 mm of the proximal edge of resection. Metastases were present in a mediastinal node.

346 Carcinoma of oesophagus (8073) Section shows transition from normal to hyperplastic squamous to dysplastic then in-situ carcinoma, and finally infiltrating keratinising squamous-cell carcinoma. *(H&E × 3)*

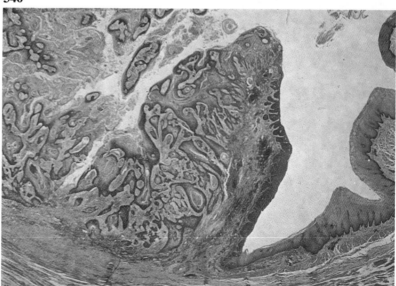

Stomach (T63)

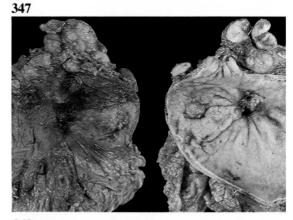

347 **Chronic peptic ulcer** (4303) from a 65-year-old woman with palpable mass and a history very suggestive of carcinoma: the specimen includes lower oesophagus and proximal half of the stomach with many enlarged nodes in both lesser and greater omentum. A 2 cm ulcer is situated on the anterior wall 2 to 3 cm from the cardia; the surrounding gastric wall feels very hard and the serosa is reddened and speckled with haemorrhages. Histologically there was no evidence of malignancy.

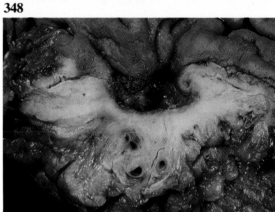

348 **Chronic peptic ulcer** (4303) from a 66-year-old man on whom a barium meal had been reported as showing carcinoma, but the lesion turned out to be a large (2.5 × 1.5 cm), deep (15 mm), chronic peptic ulcer on lesser curvature with much induration of the adjacent wall.

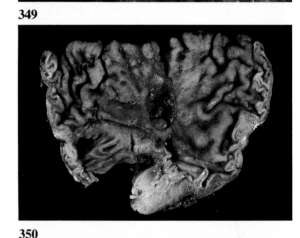

349 **Chronic peptic ulcer** (4303) on the lesser curvature of part of the stomach from 69-year-old bus driver, with history of gastroenterostomy for gastric ulcer and admitted with haematemesis. A large eroded artery is seen on the floor of the benign chronic peptic ulcer: the gastric mucosa showed marked small intestinal metaplasia and severe chronic antral gastritis was evident. The gastroenterostomy appeared intact.

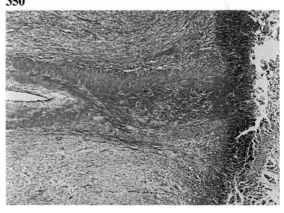

350 **Chronic peptic ulcer** (4303) A section to show chronic peptic ulcer with involved artery in the base. *(H&E × 13)*

351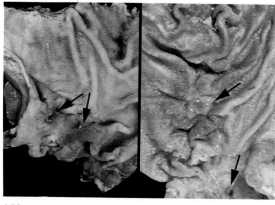

351 Multiple peptic ulcers (4300) Left shows 'kissing ulcers' (arrowed) in the antrum and right, a gastric ulcer (arrowed) just proximal to the pylorus and a duodenal ulcer (arrowed) just distal.

352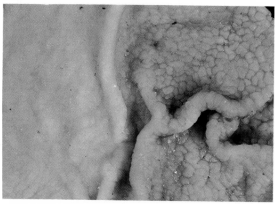

352 Chronic gastritis (etat mamellone) (4300) Partial gastrectomy was done on this 38-year-old woman with duodenal ulcer. The sleeve of the stomach was 12 cm along the greater curvature and the mucosa showed an abrupt transition from dark fine nodularity proximally to smooth pallor distally. Histologically there was focal superficial chronic gastritis.

353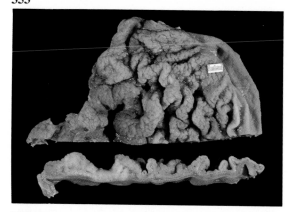

353 Hypertrophic gastritis (7242) with ulcerated carcinoma of the antrum: in the longitudinal slice cyst formation is seen in the deeper parts of the thickened mucosa, changes usually associated with Ménétrier's disease.

354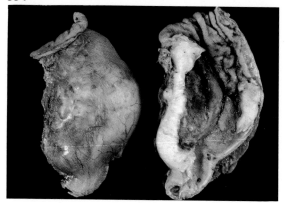

354 Anaplastic malignant round-cell neoplasm (8003) of the stomach from 59-year-old woman presenting with anaemia and epigastric mass. The serosal surface over the middle third anteriorly and most of the surface posteriorly is pale and nodular as a result of infiltration by neoplasm, which has produced a fungating ulcerated wall up to 2.5 cm thick. The neoplasm extends to the plane of excision proximally but stops in the pyloric canal, the duodenum being spared. Sections were reported as showing highly cellular (mitoses up to 20 per HP field) undifferentiated round-cell neoplasm. No agreement could be reached as to whether it was a carcinoma or a sarcoma, although most favoured the latter.

355 Poorly differentiated glandular carcinoma (8023) of the stomach from a 64-year-old man who complained of melaena, abdominal pain and flatulence. Total gastrectomy with splenectomy and partial pancreatectomy was done. Large finger-like neoplastic masses lay in lymphatics in both omenta. A very large (11 × 9 cm) ulcerated carcinoma generally of undifferentiated polyhedral-cell type with numerous and abnormal mitoses (up to 50 per HP field) penetrates the wall and extends to within 5 cm of each end of the specimen. Many nodes show replacement by metastases.

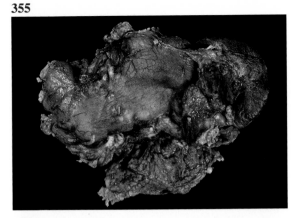

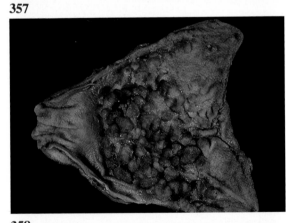

356 Carcinoma of the stomach (8023) with widespread lymphatic involvement: same specimen as in **355** showing the opened stomach with very extensive replacement of gastric wall, yet the capacity of the organ has altered little.

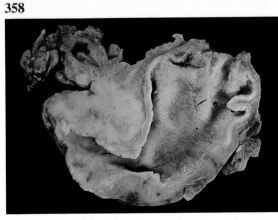

357 Multiple polyposis of the stomach (8053) with development of papillary superficial glandular carcinoma, apparently still at an early stage, from a 72-year-old hairdresser. The specimen is a segment of the stomach 14 cm long with multiple polypi (from pinhead size to 2.5 cm) studded over the mucosa from the proximal cut end to within 4.5 cm of the distal. Histologically all but two of the polypi were benign papillary adenomas: in these two the appearances were those of papillary superficial glandular carcinoma arising in cellular papillary adenomas. No enlarged nodes were found.

358 Squamous-cell carcinoma of the stomach (8073) from a 57-year-old man with obstructive jaundice and thought to have a carcinoma of pancreas, but at operation the neoplasm (4 × 3.5 × 3 cm) was situated on the lesser curvature of the stomach, the wall of which was diffusely infiltrated by well-differentiated keratinising squamous-cell carcinoma. No other primary site was found.

106

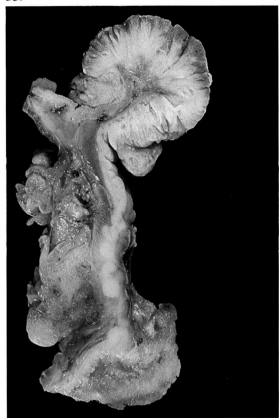

359

359 Ulcerated adenocarcinoma (8143) arising in stomach showing large (3.5 cm) adenomatous polyp at the antrum and widespread *in situ* carcinoma as well as small intestinal metaplasia.

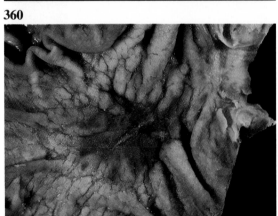

360

360 Superficial carcinoma of the stomach (8143) from a 43-year-old woman known to have Crohn's disease of the small bowel and admitted with a gastric lesion. Biopsy showed a gastric carcinoma. The lesion was a (2 × 1.5 cm) dark-reddish area of holly-leaf outline; on section it appeared confined to the mucosa. There was focal small intestinal metaplasia, a small chronic peptic ulcer and active chronic superficial gastritis, but no diagnostic evidence of Crohn's disease.

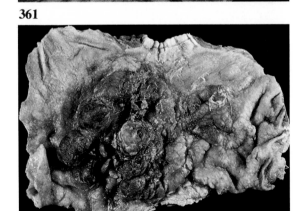

361

361 Carcinoma of the stomach (8143) from a 70-year-old man. The specimen is an 11 cm long part of the stomach with a large (10 × 8 cm) fungating haemorrhagic mass reaching from just below the gastro-oesophageal junction almost to the plane of resection. Histologically it was a glandular carcinoma with papillary pattern and it invaded the muscle coat, but did not penetrate.

362 Carcinoma of the cardia (8143) from a 48-year-old fitter's mate showing extensive infiltration of lower oesophagus and of much of the lesser curvature of the stomach, with metastases in nodes in lesser omentum. The lesion was 12cm at its widest reaching to within 5mm of the proximal edge of resection and extending to the distal resection line at one point.

363 Leather-bottle stomach, linitis plastica (8143) from a 47-year-old man. The specimen consists of a complete stomach (30cm along greater curvature) with short length of oesophagus and duodenum (3cm each) and a piece (8×3cm) of pancreas adherent to the posterior wall of the antrum. A diffuse carcinoma infiltrates the wall from gastro-oesophageal junction to within 3cm of the pylorus. Nodes on the lesser curvature are replaced by metastases. Sections show mucin-secreting glandular carcinoma (signet ring). The spleen (60g) also removed was free of neoplasm.

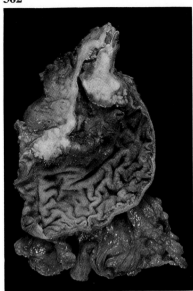

362

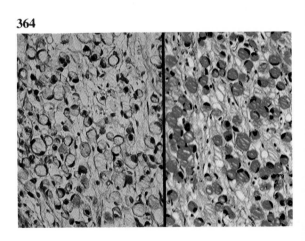

363

364

364 Leather-bottle stomach (8143) Section to show signet-ring cell carcinoma. *(H&E on left, Alcian-van Gieson on right ×83)*

365

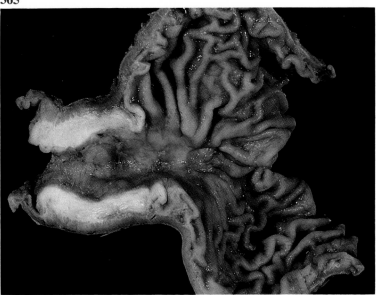

365 Carcinoma of the stomach (8143) in a 27-year-old woman with a long history of dyspepsia attributed to gastric ulcer. The specimen of stomach is 15 cm along the greater curvature, 8 cm along the lesser curvature: on the latter 3 cm from the proximal cut edge there is an ovoid chronic peptic ulcer (2 × 1 cm) and its distal margin merges into an ulcerated carcinoma involving the whole antrum, but stopping short at duodenal mucosa. The development of carcinoma in the wall of a chronic peptic ulcer takes place in only a small proportion of cases (about 1 to 2 per cent).

366

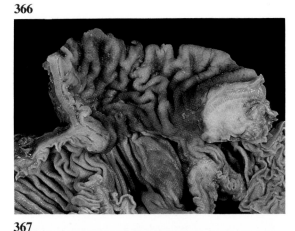

366 Carcinoma of gastric origin in gastroenterostomy stoma (8143) from a man who had a Polya-gastrectomy 20 years ago. The disc of stomach measured 10 cm in diameter and includes a (4 × 3 cm) stoma with afferent and efferent loops of jejunum. A mucin-producing carcinoma infiltrates the margin of the stoma mainly on the gastric side, and replaced several enlarged nodes in the omentum.

367

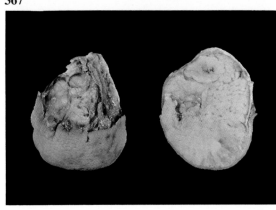

367 Carcinoid tumour of the stomach (apudoma arising in ectopic pancreas) (8240) of a woman with recurrent haematemesis – gastrotomy showed the cause to be a polypoid tumour (7 × 6 × 5 cm) with lobulated pink-grey to yellow-white cut surface. The initial report on cryostat section was that it was an unusual neoplasm with areas of carcinoid pattern (and some cells giving a positive argyrophil reaction), while others showed an acinar arrangement with mucin and zymogen granules in the cytoplasm resembling pancreas. The overlying mucosa was inflamed but intact.

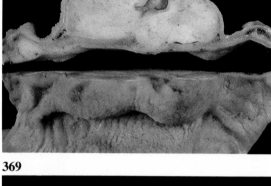
368

368 **Bizarre leiomyoblastoma of the stomach** (8890) from a 63-year-old jute worker being investigated for anaemia: faecal occult blood was persistently positive. Barium meal showed a filling defect corresponding to the umbilicated (6×4×2cm) neoplasm with greyish-pink lobulated cut surface, apparently encapsulated. Histologically it showed polyhedral cells with clear cytoplasm and giant multinucleate cells in areas of degeneration.

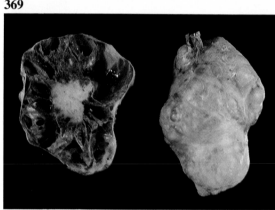
369

369 **Bizarre leiomyoblastoma of the stomach** (8890) from a 75-year-old woman. The mass is 1.3cm in diameter, weighs 625g and was attached to the gastric wall by a narrow pedicle (2.2×0.6cm).

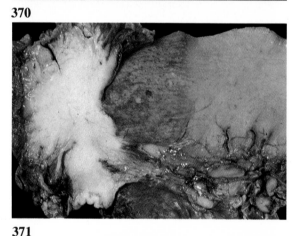
370

370 **Lymphosarcoma of the stomach** (9623) from a 42-year-old man with a short history of dyspepsia. At operation diffuse pale induration was seen beginning near the pylorus and extending proximally for 7cm. A biopsy was reported as showing diffuse lymphocytic lymphoma with a nodular pattern in some areas.

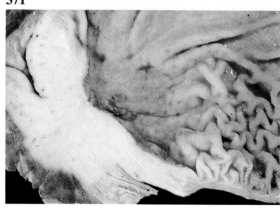
371

371 **Lymphosarcoma of the stomach** (9623) Same specimen as in **370** showing appearances after slicing away the anterior wall. The gastric rugae are thickened and pale as a result of neoplastic infiltration and there is ulceration in the antrum where the wall is several centimetres thick.

372   Hodgkin's disease of the stomach (9653) in a 65-year-old woman diagnosed 11 years earlier as having Hodgkin's disease. Admitted as an emergency – ?'perforated ulcer': the stomach had ruptured at the fundus through a large ulcerated area producing a 9 cm long tear. A (5 × 3 cm) ulcer is present in the antrum where neoplastic infiltration is also widespread. A mass of enlarged nodes (up to 2 cm) is present in the lesser omentum proximally and there are five other large nodes lower down. Histologically the sections showed infiltration of gastric wall and nodes by neoplasm of Hodgkin's type (lymphocyte depleted) with mirror-image and giant cells in some areas.

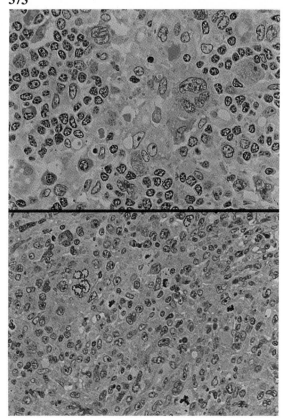

373   Hodgkin's disease of the stomach (9653) Same specimen as in **372**. Plastic sections to show mirror-image cells, giant cells (Reed-Sternberg), plasma cells and a few lymphocytes. The field below shows several mitoses including one triaster. *(Dominici × 133, × 83)*

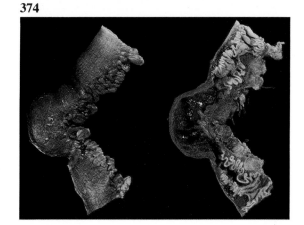

374   Richter's hernia (2810) from a femoral herniotomy on an 83-year-old woman presenting with intestinal obstruction. The partially infarcted 12 cm loop of small bowel was resected and an end-to-end anastomosis successfully achieved. The central knuckle (4 cm in length) is plum coloured and shows fibrinous exudate on its serosal surface. The sections of this area showed oedema, haemorrhage and necrosis of mucosa and part of the muscularis propria.

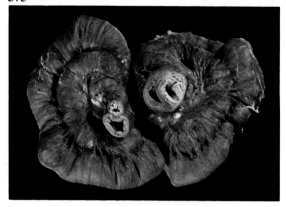 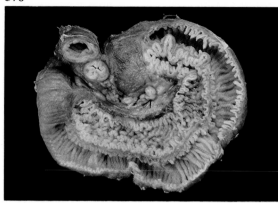

Small intestine (T64)

375 Duplication of the small intestine (2810) from a four-year-old boy presenting with gastrointestinal bleeding and a history of having had excision of peptic ulcer after perforation. At laparotomy an extensive duplication of the small bowel was resected: a 60 cm length of small intestine with mesentery in which there is tubular duplication showing a striking contrast between the thin brown villous small intestinal type mucosa of the normal 'outermost loop' and the pale rugose gastric type mucosa of the inner. The contents

of the latter had a low pH. The serosal surface is roughened because of adhesions from previous inflammation.

376 Duplication of the small intestine (2810) Part of the specimen shown in **375**. The anterior walls of the normal (outer) and duplication have been removed to demonstrate the contrasting appearance of the normal small intestinal mucosa and that of the gastric type in the duplication.

377

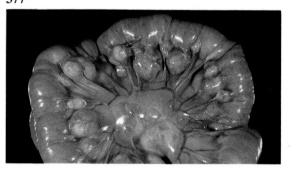

377 Jejunal diverticulosis (3476) from a 70-year-old man known to have malabsorption syndrome and who died after several haematemeses from gastric erosions: at necropsy he was shown to have diverticular disease of the duodenum and jejunum and also of the sigmoid colon. The photograph shows numerous diverticula on the mesenteric aspect of the jejunum, the wall of which is abormally brown ('brown bowel'), caused by accumulation of lipofuscin in smooth muscle cells and thought to reflect vitamin E deficiency.

378

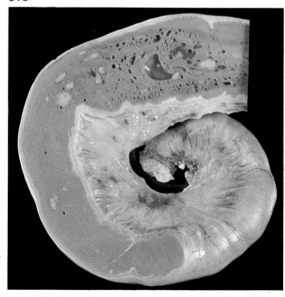

378 Meconium ileus (3509) from a two-day-old girl with fibrocystic disease of the pancreas (mucoviscidosis). Two lengths of small intestine (30 × 18 cm) were resected. They both showed gross dilatation (to a width of 3 cm) and contained firm, dry light-brown meconium. The sections confirmed that there was mucoviscidosis and that the bowel wall was viable.

379

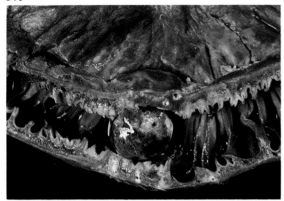

379 Gallstone ileus (3600) from an 81-year-old man presenting as an 'acute abdomen with obstruction and peritonitis'. The resected 42 cm of the ileum included a central area of intense inflammation at the site of impacted 2 cm in diameter gallstone. The stone is of mixed cholesterol and pigment type. The close-up photograph shows intense redness of serosa, green bile staining especially in some thinned areas, and abscess formation in thickened wall with ulceration adjacent to the stone. The route of entry is usually through a cholecyst-enteric fistula. Numerous other stones were present in the necrotic gallbladder.

380

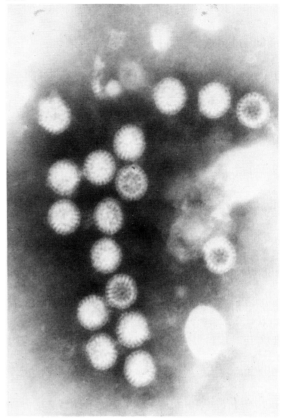

380 Electronmicrograph of Rotavirus (E 3600) from a case of gastroenteritis in a child. *(× 132,000)*

381 Ulcerative jejunitis (4003) on the left from a 67-year-old woman admitted with 'subacute obstruction'. A 10 cm length of jejunum included, at one end a 3 cm long thickened part with ulcerated mucosa and narrowed lumen, then a wider part of 2 cm, then another ulcerated stricture. Histologically the appearances were those of non-specific chronic jejunitis without tuberculoid granuloma or neoplasm. There was no history of potassium tablet ingestion and follow-up has not shown any sign of Crohn's disease or of lymphoma. On the right ulcerative ileitis with perforations from a 68-year-old man with a history of biliary peritonitis. The 18 cm length of ileum and attached mesentery showed fat necrosis with bile staining. On the antimesenteric border 4 cm from one end there was a 1 cm perforation and 5 cm from the other a large 2.5 cm defect. Large irregular ulcers (up to 4 cm in diameter) in oedematous mucosa are shown in the close-up photograph in which a probe lies in the smaller perforation (top). Histologically no clues were found as to the aetiology: in particular no arteritis, no micro-organisms and no parasites were identified and no neoplasm was present. It was felt that the disease might have been caused by an enterovirus.

381

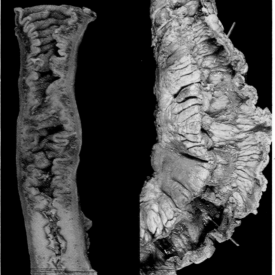

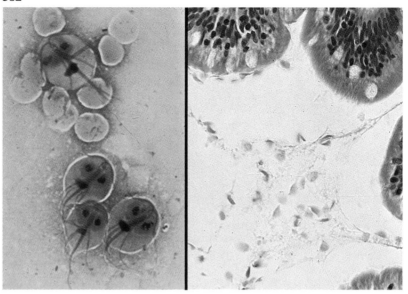

382 Giardiasis (E 4458) Imprint (on left) from jejunal biopsy from a one-year-old girl with history of failure to thrive (malabsorption syndrome). It has been stained with Giemsa's stain and shows four vegetative forms of the parasite Giardia intestinalis: the kinetoplast is seen astride the axostyles, the two nuclei lie towards the anterior end and there are four pairs of flagellae. On the right, section of jejunal biopsy from two-year-old boy with diarrhoea and thought to have coeliac disease; the biopsy showed partial villous atrophy and abundant Giardia lamblia in the crypts. In this situation one needs to treat the infestation, then repeat the biopsy if one is to resolve the problem of whether the lesions are caused by the parasite. *(×330×133)*

383

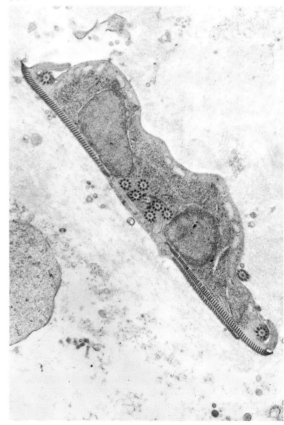

383 Giardia lamblia (E 4458) Electronmicrograph of the parasite in transverse section showing the flagella with (9 + 2) arrangement of fibrils, and the two nuclei, one on each side. *(×18,500)*

384

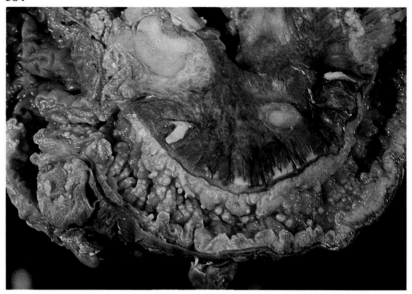

384   Ileitis with appendicitis (?viral ?yersinial) (4140) from a 10-year-old boy admitted with a history suggesting acute appendicitis. At emergency nocturnal laparotomy the operator was alarmed by the enlargement of the lymph nodes and terminal ileum and resected 22 cm of terminal ileum inflamed 5.5 cm long vermiform appendix and 9 cm of caecum. These all appeared deeply congested and there was fibrinopurulent exudate over all three, but maximal around the appendix, the distal half of which is necrotic and almost black in colour. The nodes in the ileocaecal angle are large (up to 3 cm) and the lymphoid tissues in the ileum, including Peyer's patches are markedly enlarged. Histologically there was a suppurative appendicitis with arteritis, mural necrosis and peritonitis. The sections of ileum showed marked lymphoid hyperplasia but no suppurative granulomas. Serological tests for virus, Salmonella and Yersinia were not diagnostic.

385

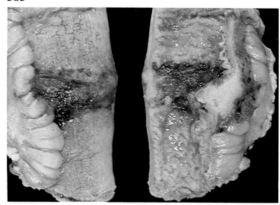

385   Tuberculous ileitis (4470) from a 20-year-old Indian student admitted with vomiting and abdominal distension of 12 hours duration. Xray showed fluid levels in small bowel. A 6 cm length of ileum including a stricture was resected. The serosal surface showed a 'transverse' band of inflammation with only two or three tubercles at the edge; the opened specimen showed narrowed lumen (from 15 to 5 mm), ulceration, and granulomatous tissue in the wall and adjacent mesentery. The histological diagnosis was confirmed by isolation of Mycobacterium tuberculosis by culture.

386

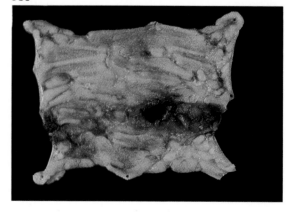

386   Acute Crohn's disease (4455) of the jejunum from a 17-year-old chef. At laparotomy the serosa was studded with tubercles and the 6 cm long piece of jejunum taken for examination showed multiple shallow irregular ulcers. Histologically the diagnosis rested between tuberculosis and acute Crohn's disease. Biopsy showed granulomatous lesions throughout the oedematous wall and on the serosa and there were 'sarcoid' lesions in lymph nodes. Lymphoid aggregates were prominent especially around inflamed dilated lymphatics. No AAFB were identified and culture for Mycobacteria was negative.

387 Subacute Crohn's disease (4455) in an unemployed 52-year-old man with signs and symptoms of intestinal obstruction, tenderness and palpable mass in right iliac fossa, and typical 'string sign of Kanter' on radiography. At laparotomy there was obvious inflammatory disease centering on the ileocaecal region. A right hemicolectomy with resection of 30cm of terminal ileum was done. The ileum lay like a letter V with three strictures and greatly thickened and ulcerated wall, the terminal 10cm of ileum being shown in the illustration. The vermiform appendix was swollen, adherent at its tip to the mesentery. The specimen was reported as severe chronic inflammation with ulcers showing pus and granulation tissue in the base, marked oedema, striking lymphoid aggregates but no tuberculoid granulomas. Mast cells and eosinophil polymorphonuclear leucocytes were very numerous and there was hypertrophy of muscle and neural elements. No parasites were identified and no neoplasm. Despite the lack of giant-cell containing lesions, the appearances were considered to be caused by Crohn's disease.

388 Chronic Crohn's disease (4455) of the terminal ileum in a 26-year-old woman. She complained of pain in the right iliac fossa (RIF) and diarrhoea, was thought to have appendicitis but at laparotomy the 'hosepipe' appearance of the terminal 7cm of the ileum was diagnosed as caused by Crohn's disease; histologically sections showed chronic ulcerative granulomatous ileitis with oedematous and fibrous thickened wall, abundant lymphoid aggregates with lymphangitis and tuberculoid granulomas in which *No* AAFB were found. Lymph nodes also showed granulomas with some giant cells containing calcium oxalate crystals (see **728**).

389 Crohn's disease (4455) with ileovesical fistula in a 75-year-old man who complained of pneumaturia and signs of small intestinal obstruction. Laparotomy revealed a fistulous communication between bladder and a thickened intensely inflamed segment of ileum beginning 6cm from the ileocaecal valve. The (2 × 1cm) piece of bladder, including the fistula, showed an unusually thickened mucosa and papillary transitional cell overgrowth.

390 Crohn's disease (4455) with ileovesical fistula: same specimen as shown in **389** opened to show thickened segment with oedematous mucosa showing deep fissures, irregular ulcers (up to 3cm wide) and small polyp formation.

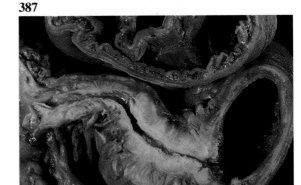

387

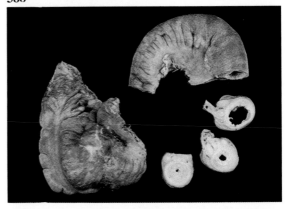

388

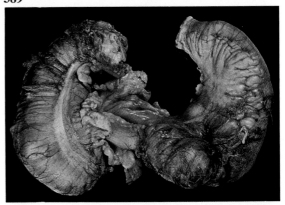

389

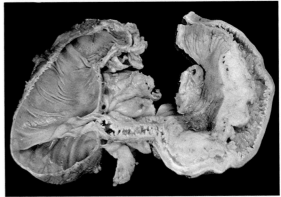

390

391 **Crohn's disease** (4455) of the terminal ileum with fistulae between loops of jejunum and ileum from a 23-year-old female with a six-month history of abdominal discomfort and two episodes of obstruction. The specimen is 40cm of ileum and 12cm of proximal large bowel. The most proximal 8cm of ileum form a V-bend, the next 18cm are dilated (up to 9cm wide), and distally make a fistulous communication with a 17cm loop of jejunum. The terminal 6cm of the ileum are narrowed (2cm) with thickened wall and cobblestone pattern mucosa. Enlarged nodes were present in the mesentery. Histologically the appearances were typical of Crohn's disease. The photograph shows the opened specimen with a probe in the fistula between adjacent loops of the ileum.

391

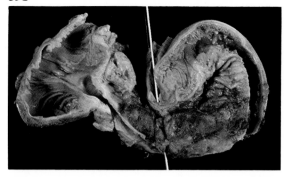

392

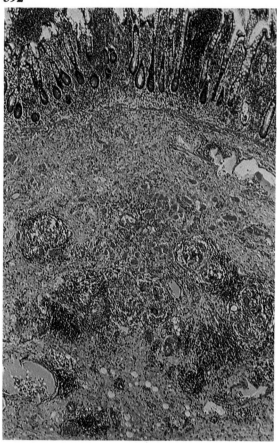

392 **Crohn's disease** (4455) of the terminal ileum. Section to show chronic inflammation of mucosa, marked submucosal oedema and lymphangitis with granulomatous foci and lymphoid aggregates. *(H&E × 13)*

393

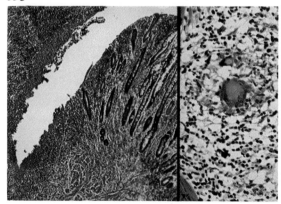

393 **Crohn's disease** (4455) of the terminal ileum. Section to show fissure with suppuration in the wall. Inset a granulomatous lesion from the muscle coat and subserosa showing multinucleate giant cells, epithelioid cells, lymphocytes, plasma cells, eosinophil polymorphs and mast cells. *(H&E × 33 × 83)*

394 Diverticulitis of the ileum (4641) from 41-year-old woman with a history suggesting acute appendicitis. The appendix was normal but 3 feet from the valve on the mesenteric border there was a fluctuant swelling (2cm in diameter), showing intense congestion and accumulation of fibrinopurulent exudate. On the cut surface the inflamed diverticulum was bilocular and communicated with the lumen through a narrow channel, the mucosa adjacent to the lesion being markedly oedematous and the muscle coat showing some hypertrophy. *No* evidence of tuberculosis, Crohn's disease or malignancy was seen; *no* amoebae were identified.

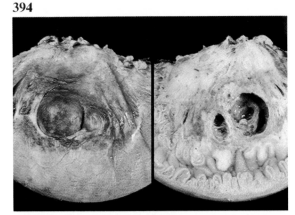

395 Post-appendicectomy infarction (5470) of the ileum from a 32-year-old machine operator who had had an appendicectomy eight weeks before; he was admitted in a state of shock with suspected pelvic abscess but at laparotomy showed an infarction of 40cm of the ileum. Interference with venous return through internal herniation or by adhesions were the two pathogenetic mechanisms thought most likely. Photograph shows abrupt transition from the normal to the infarcted dark plum-coloured bowel.

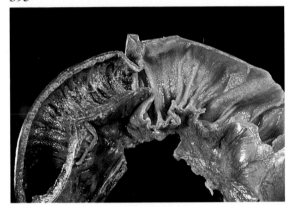

396 Peutz-Jeghers polyp (5747) of the jejunum with malignant change in a 34-year-old Irishman with intestinal obstruction. He had numerous small pigmented areas on his lips and was cachectic. At laparotomy a jejuno-jejunal intussusception with a polypoid mass at its apex was resected. The specimen was a 9cm length of jejunum with a centrally placed 3cm diameter polyp with indurated base. Histologically the lesion was reported as glandular carcinoma arising in a hamartomatous polyp with an unusual complement of mucin-secreting cells, Paneth cells, and Kulchitsky cells intermingled with columnar and cuboidal cells supported on papillary processes of fibrous and muscular tissue. In places acini resembling Brunner's glands were noted and the carcinomatous areas showed cells with deeply basophilic cytoplasm. A lymph node from the related mesentery contained metastatic carcinoma. *(H&E × 1.5)*

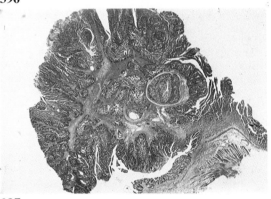

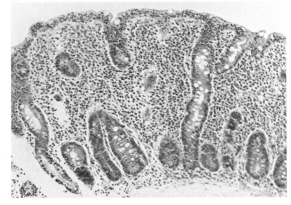

397 Jejunal villous atrophy (7100) (flat mucosa) in coeliac disease. Histologically the villous atrophy is associated with a chronic jejunitis and an increase in the number of lymphocyte nuclei in the surface and glandular epithelium. *(H&E × 53)*

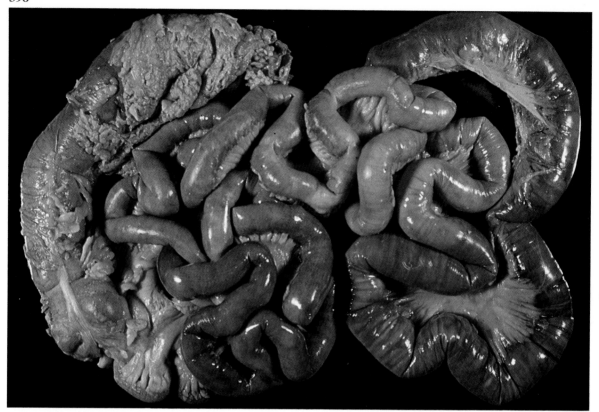

398 Mesenteric embolism (3710) with infarction of all but 6cm of the small bowel from a 74-year-old retired plater who was known to have atrial fibrillation and presented with sudden abdominal pain and passing of fresh red blood in the stool. The specimen comprises 400cm of small bowel with ileocaecal valve and proximal 46cm of caecum and ascending colon. The proximal 90cm of jejunum is dilated (5.5cm diameter) and dark red, changing abruptly to a narrower (4cm) paler loop for 135cm. Then there is a slight change in colour and calibre (3cm) for 30cm with another dilated (4cm) darker red swollen loop for 135cm. The terminal 15cm of the ileum appears normal, while the caecum and colon are 7cm wide and congested. The lumens of two major ileal arteries were occluded by recent thromboembolus. Histologically the appearances were those of recent infarction with early peritonitis. The vermiform appendix (7cm) showed appearance of chronic appendicitis with a focus of recent intramural suppuration near the tip.

399 Whipple's disease (5504) Jejunal biopsy from a 42-year-old man with multisystem disease including arthritis, pneumonitis, pericarditis, haematuria and steatorrhoea. He had a continuing pyrexia and raised ESR as well as a positive RA latex test. The initial biopsy was reported as showing a highly abnormal mucosa with partial villous atrophy, crypt hyperplasia, focal acute inflammation, and numerous mononuclear cells with PAS-positive granules in their cytoplasm. Electronmicrographs (see **400**) showed diagnostic bacilliform bodies. After treatment a repeat biopsy showed near normal villous pattern, but persistence of the mononuclear cells in the deeper lamina propria. *(H&E and PAS-H × 133)*

400 Whipple's disease (5504) Electronmicrograph of the biopsy shown in **399** to show bacilliform bodies, on the right in transverse section, on the left longitudinal. *(× 30,000)*

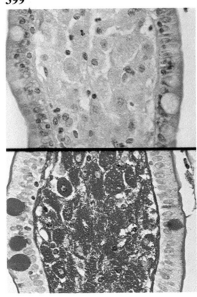

399

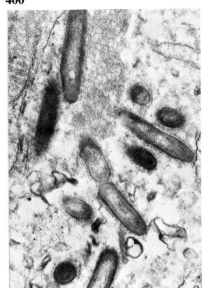

400

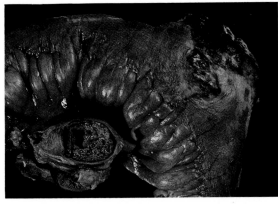

401

401 Metastatic carcinoma (8016) (malignant melanoma) in the jejunum. Primary carcinoma of the small bowel is uncommon, so that one should always think of the possibility of metastases or malignant lymphoma when faced with a malignant tumour of the small bowel. Among the extra-abdominal primary lesions malignant melanoma and thyroid carcinoma are the most common. Intra-abdominal primary lesions would include colon, stomach, ovary or uterus (cervical carcinoma or chorioncarcinoma).

Small intestine (T64)

402a Ampullary carcinoma (8143) from a 58-year-old domestic servant who presented with increasing jaundice caused by an obstructive lesion of the common bile duct. A Whipple's operation produced distal 10cm of stomach and duodenum with a 6×6×2cm part of pancreas and accompanying lymph nodes, four containing metastatic neoplasm. The dilated (up to 2.6cm) common bile duct narrows at its lower end, where a solid and papillary carcinoma replaces the ampulla of Vater forming a mass 2.5×2cm. No adenomas are seen on the rest of the mucosa. Histologically the lesion was a well-differentiated glandular carcinoma.

402b Ampullary carcinoma (8143) from a 54-year-old man with obstructive jaundice due to a large (5cm) papillary adenocarcinoma of the ampulla of Vater.

403 Intussusception of ileoileal type (8143) caused by ileal carcinoma from an adult woman known to have malabsorption syndrome, and presenting with persistent vomiting. At operation invagination of the ileum into the part below was apparent and the intussusceptum could not be wholly removed from the intussuscipiens: a 12cm length of intestine was removed including a circumferential white neoplasm 3cm long causing obstruction and forming the apex of the intussusception. In children it is unusual to find such an obvious cause as a tumour at the apex of the intussusception, though hyperplastic lymphoid tissue associated with adenovirus infection, or hamartoma such as a Meckel's diverticulum may be responsible.

404 Carcinoid tumour of ileum (8243) from an 84-year-old man with intestinal obstruction: 30cm of ileum were resected: 12cm from one end there is an indrawing of the wall, the bowel proximally being dilated.

405 Carcinoid tumour of ileum (8243) Same specimen as in **404** to show opened ileum with *two* lesions. The larger (3×2cm) obstructive lesion shows the typical yellow colour of carcinoid tumour and also the eccentric thickening of the wall at the site of the lesion. The smaller (1.0×1.0cm) tumour (arrowed) near the other end is also yellow and the mucosa over it has become ulcerated. It is common for carcinoid tumours in the ileum to be multiple – as many as nine have been seen in a specimen in our collection. There were four enlarged nodes, two of which showed metastases.

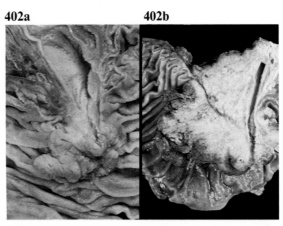

402a   402b

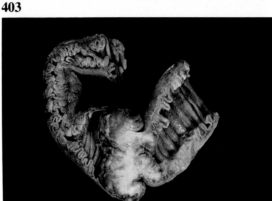

403

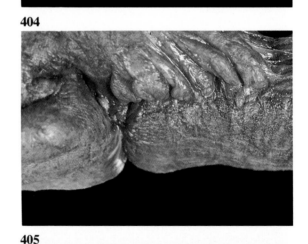

404

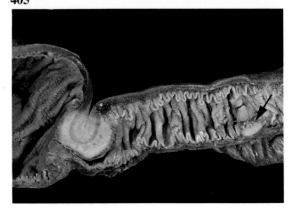

405

406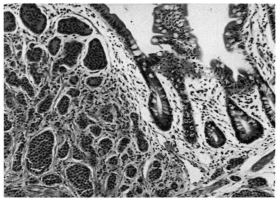

407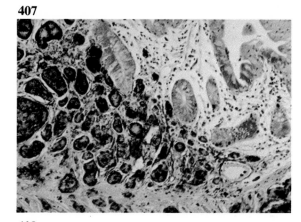

408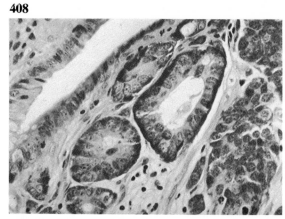

406 Carcinoid tumour of ileum (8243) Section from edge of lesion showing characteristic alveolar arrangement of polyhedral cells with uniform round nuclei and cytoplasm which stains with eosin, but often shows a faint brownish granularity particularly towards the periphery of masses of neoplasm: lumen formation may occur: mitotic activity is usually not great but infiltration and penetration of wall is usual. Desmoplasia and elastosis are variable but may be quite striking. *(H&E × 53)*

407 Carcinoid tumour of ileum (8243) Same specimen as in **406** stained with silver method (diamine silver) to demonstrate argentaffinity. Note the presence of Kulchitsky cells (stained black) in the crypts and how the silver reaction is more pronounced towards the periphery of the neoplastic masses. *(× 53)*

408 Carcinoid tumour of ileum (8243) Section to show cytoplasmic granules stained with Haematoxylin Phloxine Degrease Lissamine Flavine. Note the Kulchitsky cell (top left) in the mucosal surface epithelium. *(× 133)*

409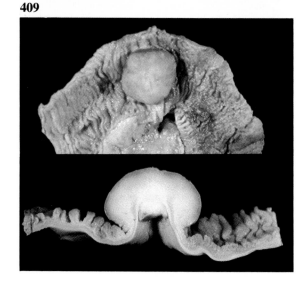

409 Leiomyoma of jejunum (8890) from a young boy presenting with intestinal obstruction. The lesion is 2.2 cm diameter and up to 1.5 cm deep and invaginates the muscle coat.

410 Perforated small bowel (9613) caused by malignant lymphoma in a 60-year-old woman suffering from a haemolytic anaemia (Coombs' test positive) and being treated with steroids. At emergency laparotomy two perforations through pale plaques were observed; after cryostat section had been reported as malignant lymphoma, 80cm of bowel and mesentery containing enlarged nodes were resected. On the left, serosal aspect of length of bowel shows the lymphomatous plaques with perforations. On the right, close-up of mucosal aspect of largest lesion (6×3cm) with (9×6mm) perforation.

411 Malignant lymphoma of small bowel (9613) from a 55-year-old man diagnosed clinically as carcinoma and treated by resection of 75cm of bowel with two discrete tumours in the wall and a large mass of nodes. A small lymphomatous nodule was present in the liver.

412 Malignant lymphoma of ileocaecal region (9613) from a 37-year-old man with history of having had treatment with radiotherapy for lymphoepithelioma of supraglottic region two years earlier. He had a peculiar diet, living solely on corn-beef sandwiches and presented with scurvy and a large abdominal mass. Hemicolectomy produced 14cm of terminal ileum and caecum and colon to a length of 18cm. The last 9cm of the ileum, and whole of caecum (9cm) from its base to its upper limit are widely infiltrated by pale, soft to firm, pink neoplasm thickening the wall (3cm) and involving serosa and ileocaecal nodes. The histological report was of malignant histiocytic lymphoma, corroborated by electronmicrography which showed no evidence of epithelial origin and immunoperoxidase preparations in which neoplastic cells appeared to contain immuno-globulins. Omentum and liver were involved.

Appendix (T66)

413 Acute suppurative appendicitis (4140) Three examples 7cm, 4cm, and 6cm long showing local peritonitis: from patients (aged 8, 12 and 34 years respectively) presenting with initial central abdominal pain and vomiting followed by pain in the RIF. The photograph shows fibrinopurulent exudate and congested vessels on the serosal surface. In each case the lumen contained pus and focal suppuration was present in the wall deep to the areas of local peritonitis. The appendix on the right also contained a faecal concretion at the tip. In the younger patients the lymphoid tissue appeared hyperplastic.

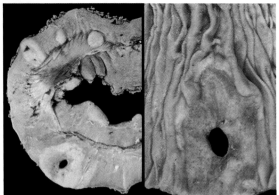

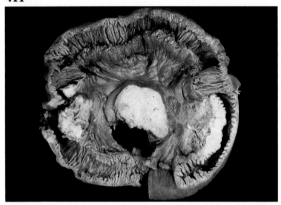

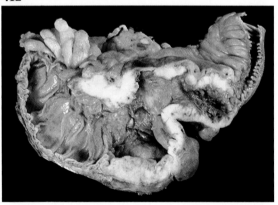

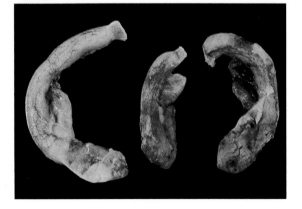

414 Acute suppurative appendicitis (4140) with obstruction of the lumen by a faecal concretion from a seven-year-old boy with a 24-hour history of abdominal pain and vomiting and with leucocytosis. The 12 cm long dilated vermiform appendix shows peritoneal exudate over all but the distal 2.5 cm which appears very congested.

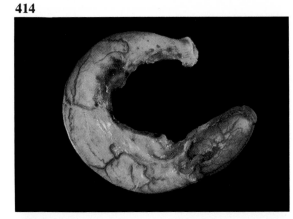

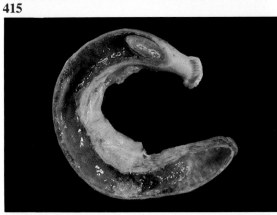

415 Acute suppurative appendicitis (4140) Same specimen as in **414** to show 15 × 6 mm ovoid faecal concretion impacted near the proximal end. The dilated lumen contained foul-smelling pus and the mucosa shows widespread ulceration.

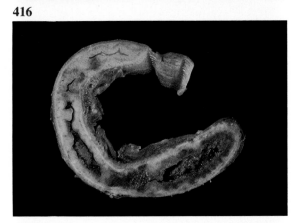

416 Acute suppurative appendicitis (4140) from a 16-year-old boy with a short (12 hour) history of central abdominal pain followed by pain in the RIF. The 10 cm long vermiform appendix is diffusely swollen and its serosa acutely inflamed. The cut surface shows lymphoid hyperplasia with narrowed lumen: the mucosa of the distal half appears red-brown and patchily ulcerated. Sections confirmed the clinical diagnosis of acute suppurative appendicitis with early peritonitis.

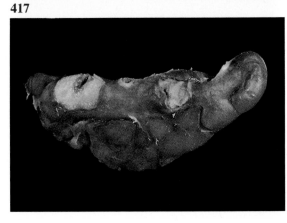

417 Perforated appendix (4140) from a 56-year-old woman presenting with a mass in the RIF. The specimen is 5.5 cm long: 15 mm from the proximal end, on the anti-mesoappendicular border, there is a (6 × 2 mm) perforation: 8 mm further on a (2 × 1 mm) perforation, and 8 mm beyond that a third (2 × 1 mm). Sections were reported as showing acute suppurative appendicitis with abscess formation leading to perforation and purulent peritonitis.

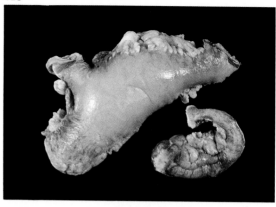

418 Acute suppurative appendicitis (4140) **and Meckel's diverticulum** (2337) removed at time of appendicectomy from an 18-year-old clerk. The 9 cm long vermiform appendix is distended and covered with fibrinopurulent exudate: its lumen contained pus and two faecal concretions. The 12 cm length of terminal ileum has a 3 × 2 cm diverticulum projecting from the antimesenteric border. Sections showed an intact ileal-type mucosa and there were no pancreatic or other heterotopic glandular tissues in the wall. Apart from serosal congestion no evidence of diverticulitis was present.

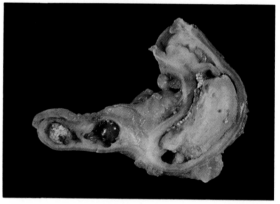

419 Acute suppurative appendicitis (4140) Section to show typical mural suppurative lesions in the mucosa and submucosa and escape of purulent exudate into the lumen, from several sites. There is extension of the inflammatory exudate into the muscle coat and on to serosa. *(H&E×2)*

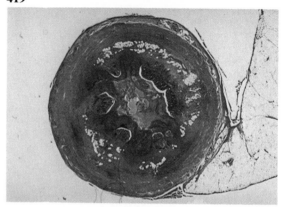

420 Chronic appendicitis with concretions (4300) A 36-year-old man's appendix removed at elective laparotomy. The 9 cm long appendix is greatly swollen (2.5 cm in diameter) over the middle third, where there is a stony hard saddle-shaped concretion (3.2 × 2.5 × 1.5 cm) impacted in the lumen. Proximally the specimen is 2 cm diameter and the lumen contained faeces: distally two smaller dark-brown concretions more or less filled the lumen and the wall is thickened and fibrous. Sections were reported as showing chronic appendicitis with widespread fibrosis of the wall and recent suppuration and ulceration adjacent to the large concretion.

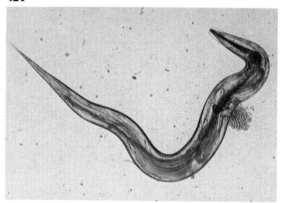

421 Enterobius vermicularis (threadworm) (E 4556) An unstained gravid female threadworm submitted for identification. It shows two alae at the head end, a double bulb oesophagus, and is discharging eggs of characteristic shape. *(×5)*

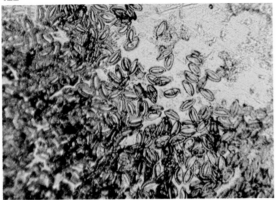

422

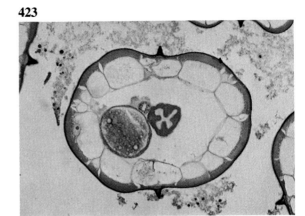

423

422 Eggs of *Enterobius vermicularis* (E 4556) collected on cellophane anal swab. They show flattening on one side and convex surface on the other. *(×83)*

423 **Enterobius vermicularis (threadworm)** (E 4556) in the lumen of a vermiform appendix removed from a young girl with symptoms suggestive of mild appen-

dicitis. The lumen contained hundreds of worms of which this is one shown in transverse section with the pathognomonic lateral cuticular spine stained green using Alcian. In semi-serial sections granulomatous lesions were found in the submucosa (see **424**). *(Alcian Phloxine × 133)*

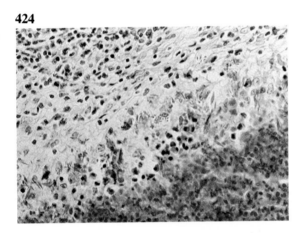

424

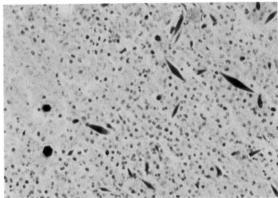

425

424 **Threadworm granuloma** (4400) in the wall of the vermiform appendix showing formation of Charcot-Leyden crystals from breakdown of the many eosinophil polymorphonuclear leucocytes in the lesion. *(H&E × 133)*

425 **Threadworm granuloma** (4400) in the wall of the vermiform appendix showing Charcot-Leyden crystals: they are hexagonal in transverse section and diamond shaped in long axis. They have been stained using a modified Giemsa's stain. *(× 133)*

426 **Trichuris trichiura (whipworm)** (E 4513) in the vermiform appendix of a Sri Lankan child who complained of abdominal pain with diarrhoea: the faeces contained typical brown barrel-shaped eggs (50 × 25 microns). Section shows the anterior narrow segment beneath the epithelium. The worm usually inhabits the caecum. *(H&E × 33)*

426

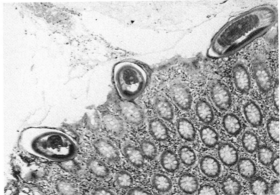

427 Spirochaetosis of the vermiform appendix (E 1800) from an 82-year-old man with symptoms suggestive of appendicitis, but the 9cm-long vermiform appendix was of normal appearance macroscopically. It was blocked in 17 pieces and no suppuration or other inflammatory process identified. The one histological feature of note, shown here, is the presence in many sections on the mucosal surface of a basophil brush-like border – appearances attributed to spirochaetal infestation. *(H&E × 133)*

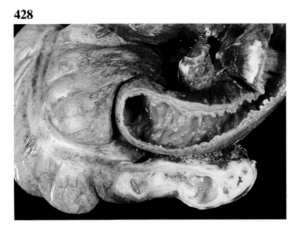

428 Carcinoma of the vermiform appendix (8143) from a 22-year-old female hairdresser with a five-day history of pain in the RIF with rebound tenderness. The specimen consisted of terminal ileum (62cm), ileocaecal valve and caecum (11cm) with 6cm long vermiform appendix distended to 3.5cm, covered with fibrinopurulent exudate and filled with pus, from which a mixed growth of Escherichia coli and anaerobic streptococci was obtained. Near the middle, the appendicular wall is largely replaced by mucoid annular neoplasm which reduces the lumen to less than 1mm. Sections showed appearances of acute suppurative appendicitis with peritonitis distal to a well-differentiated mucin-secreting (in places signet ring) glandular carcinoma, which infiltrated muscularis propria without penetrating it. Carcinomatous cells were present in lymphatics, but no metastases were seen in sections at many levels of the enlarged nodes in the ileocaecal angle.

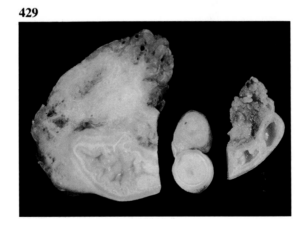

429 Appendix abscess with carcinoid tumour (8240) from a 19-year-old youth. The specimen was a 6cm-long vermiform appendix with swollen distal 2cm adherent to a 5×5×3cm fibrofatty mass containing small abscess cavities. On section, the distal part shows a dilated lumen with a diverticulum passing through hypertrophied muscle coat: near the centre of the specimen the lumen is obstructed by a yellow solid neoplasm, histologically a carcinoid tumour. Acute and chronic inflammatory changes were present in the wall of the appendix.

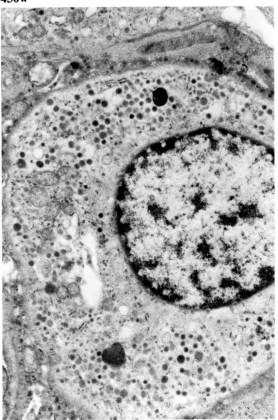

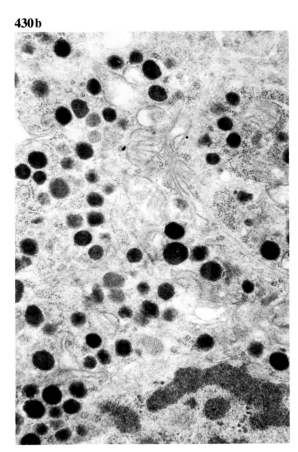

430a & 430b   Carcinoid tumour of vermiform appendix (8240) Same lesion as **429**. Electronmicrographs to show intracytoplasmic neurosecretory spherical (membrane bound) granules of variable size with electron-dense core. *(×7,000) (×24,000)*

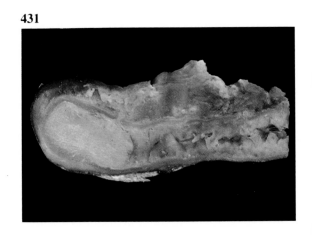

431   Carcinoid tumour of the vermiform appendix (8240) from a young woman with symptoms of pelvic inflammation. At laparotomy a 6cm-long vermiform appendix with bulbous tip (1.3cm) caused by a circumscribed yellow tumour (12×6mm) was removed. Histologically it infiltrated the whole thickness of the wall invading mesoappendicular fat. No evidence of appendicitis was found, but the fallopian tube removed at the same time showed suppurative salpingitis.

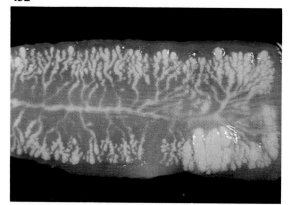

432 **Tapeworm (segment of Taenia saginata)** (E 4715) from a butcher who admitted eating raw sausages. The segment, one of many single proglottides submitted for identification, was 2 × 1 cm. The photograph shows the numerous dichotomous branches of the gravid uterus.

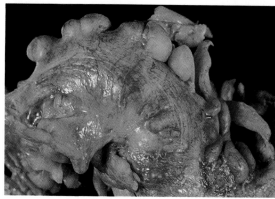

433 **Diverticulosis coli** (3476) in a 77-year-old man with diarrhoea off and on for one year, recent melaena and weight loss and suspected as carcinoma, but the 18 cm length of the sigmoid colon showed multiple diverticula with some of them inflamed and one related to a pericolic abscess. The close-up shows diverticula on either side of the taenia and enlarged appendices epiploicae. No carcinoma was found.

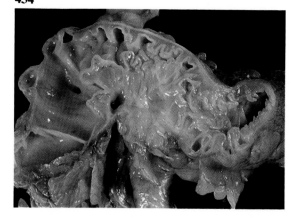

434 **Diverticulosis coli** (3476) Same lesion as in **433** sliced longitudinally to show greatly hypertrophied muscle coat, multiple diverticula, the one left of centre showing reddened inflamed lining, and the adjacent mesocolon and colon showing fibrous scarring.

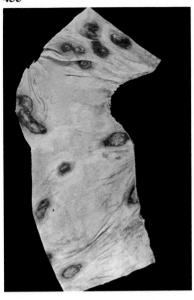

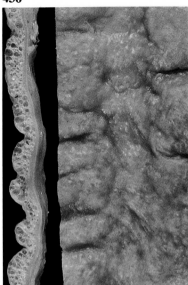

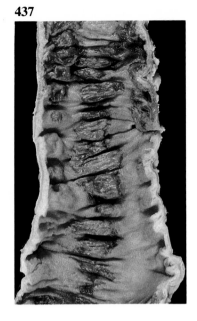

Large intestine (T67 and T68)

435   Colonic mucosal infarction (5470) in polyarteritis nodosa complicated by opportunistic fungal (aspergillus) infection after treatment with steroids.

436   Pneumatosis coli (3570) complicating carcinoma of the colon after its removal by hemicolectomy. Bubbles of gas are seen throughout the mucosa and submucosa and histologically a characteristic wall of multinucleate macrophages accumulates around the gas. Eventually the gas is absorbed and the whole process resolves.

437   Mucosal infarction in DIC (5470) (disseminated intravascular coagulation) complicating tertian malaria in a ship's captain.

438   Uraemic colitis (4057) **and melanosis coli** (5711) in a 48-year-old woman in renal failure caused by bilateral hydronephrosis. There was excess mucus secretion, mucosal hyperaemia and oedema with a few small superficial ulcers.

439   Pseudomembranous colitis (4055) in a 78-year-old man on antibiotics for chronic pulmonary fibrosis with bronchiectasis. The patchy membrane consists of fibrinous and purulent exudate with desquamated epithelial cells; on culture a pure growth of Clostridium difficile was obtained.

440   Amoebic colitis (4000) from a 70-year-old Scotswoman who had never been abroad and was thought to have a malignant disease. There were typical flask-shaped pits in the rectum, and larger irregular sloughing ulcers in the sigmoid, transverse and ascending colons.

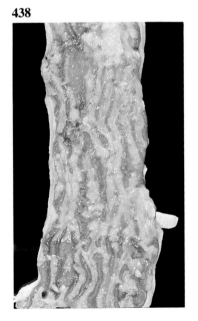

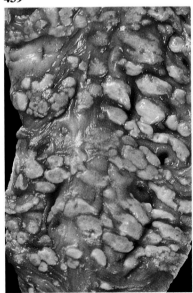

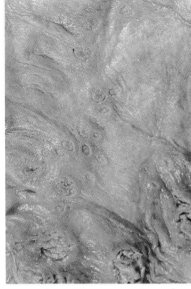

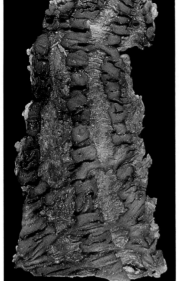

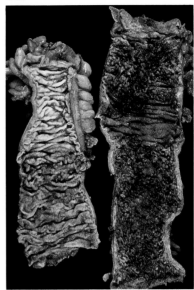

441 Ulcerative colitis (4003) from a 66-year-old chartered accountant with an eight-week history of diarrhoea with blood and mucus in stools and associated with marked weight loss. Sigmoidoscopy showed irregular granular rectal mucosa but ulceration of the sigmoid. Total colectomy was done. The specimen shows longitudinal confluent ulcers bordered by overhanging mucosa showing intense congestion and inflammation (see **448** and **449**).

442 Granulomatous colitis (4455) with pseudopolyposis from a 54-year-old man with a 13-year history of chronic inflammatory bowel disease, culminating in a resection of a carcinoma of the transverse colon. Nine months later two further pieces of the colon 20 cm and 15.5 cm respectively were excised and these were reported as showing inflammatory pseudopolyposis with bridging and branching (well recognised as

occurring in Crohn's disease) and granulomatous reaction including follicular lesions with multinucleate giant cells, and *no* AAFB. Here the macroscopic and microscopic appearances seemed to fit Crohn's disease, yet some pathologists felt that it was a form of ulcerative colitis.

443 Ulcerative colitis (4003) with polyposis and stricture distal to splenic flexure from a 70-year-old man treated by total colectomy. The 110 cm of the colon showed widespread congestion and ulceration with a 6 cm-long stricture close to an area showing cobblestone pattern with ulceration between projecting mucosal mounds. In this case no granulomatous lesions were present and the process affected mainly mucosa and submucosa, so that it was reported as a form of ulcerative colitis. The terminal ileum was not inflamed.

443 **444**

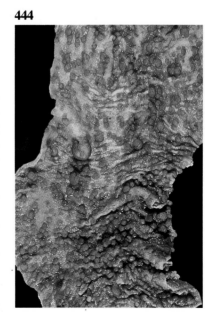

444 Polyposis coli (8220) from a 30-year-old nurse with a carcinoma of the rectum (see **489**). The whole of the colon is studded with polypoid adenomas ranging in size from a pinhead to 2 cm.

445

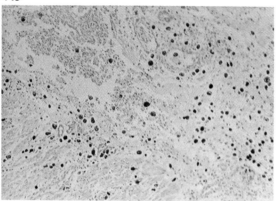

446

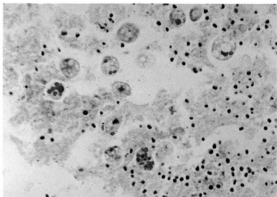

447

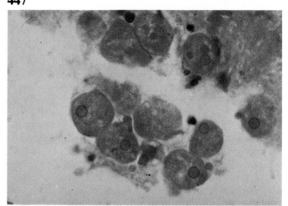

445 Amoebic colitis (4000) in a section of colonic ulcer with undermined edge in which vast numbers of PAS-positive amoebae are demonstrable. Examination of exudate from the ulcer edge on a warm stage showed diagnostic Entamoeba histolytica. *(PAS×33)*

446 Amoebiasis (7763) Section stained to show Entamoeba histolytica with ingested erythrocytes (same case as **13**). *(KRAG ×83)*

447 Amoebiasis (E 4422) Section of a rectal biopsy from a 37-year-old woman thought to have ulcerative colitis. In the mucus and blood accompanying chronically inflamed rectal mucosal fragments there are many Entamoeba histolytica, identified by their central karyosome, delicate chromatin on the nuclear membrane, and by erythrophagy. *(H&E×330)*

448

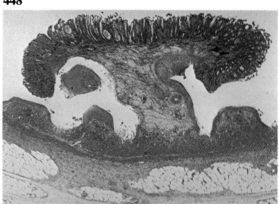

449

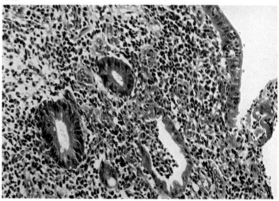

448 Ulcerative colitis (4003) Section from the case shown in **441** to show mucosal inflammation with ulceration: dilated crypts contain pus, which is also present in the ulcer base and undermined edge. The inner layer of muscle coat shows some involvement by chronic inflammation. *(H&E×2.5)*

449 Ulcerative colitis (4003) Section from same case as in **441** to show crypt abscess and dense chronic inflammatory cell infiltration of lamina propria. *(H&E×53)*

450

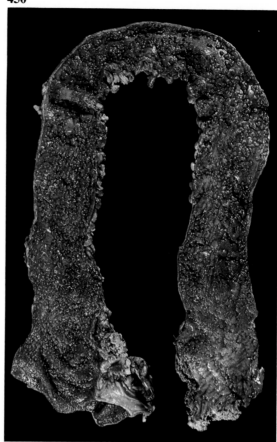

450 Ulcerative colitis (4003) in a 13½-year-old boy with up to 20 motions a day, abdominal pain, weightloss and no response to steroids. There is widespread ulceration and surviving mucosa shows congestion and tendency to polypoid hyperplasia. The rectum appears less severely affected than the rest of colon while the ileum (bottom left) is not involved.

451

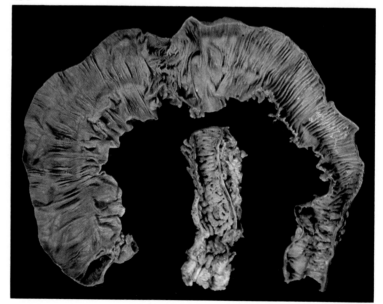

451 Ulcerative colitis (4003) in a 30-year-old man with a two-month history of diarrhoea, and passing blood and mucus. At panproctocolectomy fistulae were noted. In the absence of lymphoid aggregates and follicular granulomas the preferred diagnosis was ulcerative colitis. Photograph shows the 120 cm of the colon with dilated proximal part: ulceration begins in the descending colon, is more severe in the sigmoid and worst in the rectum.

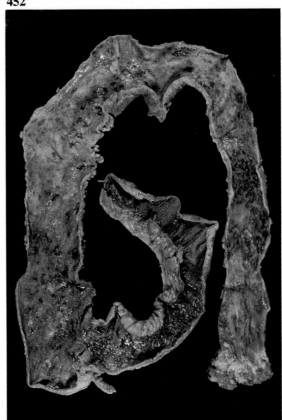

452 **Ulcerative colitis** (4003) with backwash terminal ileitis in a woman with a long history of diarrhoea. The colectomy specimen measures 90cm from anus to ileocaecal valve; 26cm of the terminal ileum shows inflamed mucosa. The 6cm vermiform appendix has an obliterated lumen. The whole of the colon and rectum shows ulcerated areas. A (3×2cm) deep ulcer in the ascending colon, a (4×2cm) superficial ulcer in the transverse colon and an irregular area of confluent ulcers (5×4cm) in the pelvic colon is visible. Between them there are numerous smaller irregular ulcers. The wall is not markedly thickened save for a 10cm length of descending and sigmoid colon. Fleshy nodes were present in the ileocaecal angle. Histologically sections showed chronic inflammation of mucosa and sub-mucosa, with granulation tissue forming pseudopolypi and without granulomas, parasites or evidence of malignancy.

453

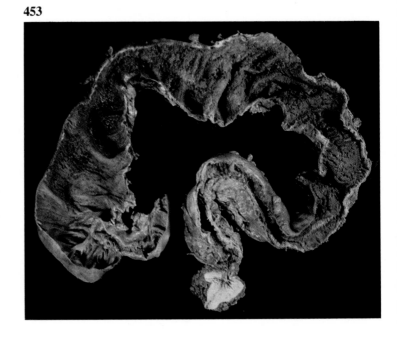

453 **Ulcerative colitis** (4003) in a 27-year-old man, with toxic megacolon, removed at abdominoperineal resection. The specimen comprises terminal 20cm of normal looking ileum and 140cm of colon and rectum. The mucosa of rectum is not severely abnormal but the rest of colonic mucosa shows intense hyperaemia with severe erosions, ulceration and pseudopolyposis but without neoplasm. Microscopy confirmed the above: frank suppuration was less prominent than seemed likely from the naked eye appearances.

454 Ulcerative colitis (4003) Total colectomy specimen showing 'regional' ulceration in ascending colon, transverse colon and sigmoid, and at anorectal junction.

454

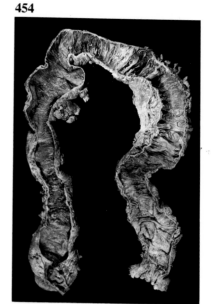

455

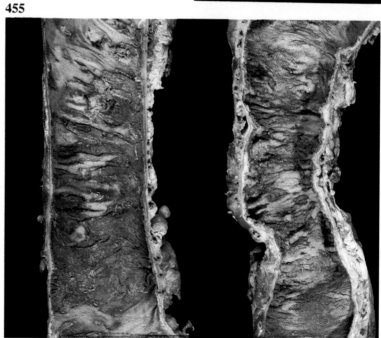

455 Ulcerative colitis (4003) on left close up of ascending colon and on right close up of transverse colon. Same specimen as **454**.

456

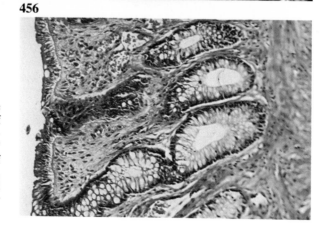

456 'Solitary ulcer of rectum' (4003) Biopsy of the rectum from a 30-year-old woman with a long history of discomfort, diarrhoea and straining at stool. At sigmoidoscopy the mucosa appeared inflamed and 'lumpy' and section of the biopsy shows typical obliteration of the lamina propria by fibrous and smooth muscle cells, and some crypt irregularity. Often a history of rectal prolapse or trauma is present and there may be no ulcer or more than one. *(H&E × 83)*

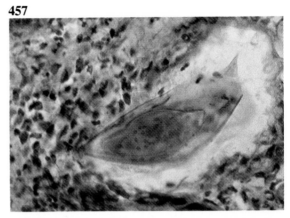

457 Schistosomiasis (4400) Rectal biopsy from a 30-year-old Kenyan Asian who complained of abdominal pain. At sigmoidoscopy the rectal mucosa appeared inflamed. Cryostat section of a biopsy was requested because it was feared that the rectum might have been perforated. The section showed only mucosa and submucosa without muscularis propria or serosa, but there were granulomatous lesions containing well preserved Schistosoma mansoni eggs with subterminal spine. *(H&E × 133)*

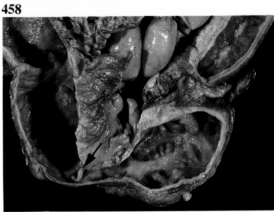

458 Crohn's disease of the ileum and colon (4455) in a 26-year-old man treated for three years with steroids. The specimen consisted of 55 cm of ileum greatly thickened in its last 9 cm, with a Meckel's diverticulum situated 35 cm from the ileocaecal valve, and 45 cm of colon showing strictures in the caecum, the mucosa of which shows finger-like polyps up to 3 cm long and up to 1 cm wide, while a bridge (arrowed) is formed by a 2 cm long narrow mucosal band. Histologically the appearances were those of a chronic enterocolitis without granulomas but otherwise consistent with Crohn's disease of the ileum and colon.

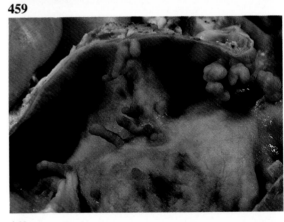

459 Crohn's disease of the colon (4455) Same lesion as in **458**. Close-up to show peniform polyps on caecal mucosa.

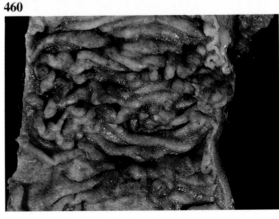

460 Granulomatous colitis: (Crohn's disease) (4455) from a 29-year-old woman diagnosed as having Crohn's disease of the rectum and buccal mucosa. After proctocolectomy she developed toxic symptoms and bled from the colostomy. A total colectomy was done. There was 10 cm of terminal ileum showing typical changes of Crohn's disease and 50 cm of the colon with areas of ulceration and polypoid mucosal hyperplasia. Mesocolonic lymph nodes showed non-caseating tuberculoid granulomas. Close-up to show swollen mucosa and pseudopolyposis.

461 **Segmented regional colitis** (4455) in a 41-year-old woman with ulcerative colitis complicated by small-bowel fistula and suspected of having Crohn's disease. But histological examination of the inflamed colon and numerous enlarged nodes showed no granulomas: the essential lesions were ulceration with suppuration on the surface of granulation tissue and crypt abscess formation, increased plasma cells in the lamina propria and melanosis.

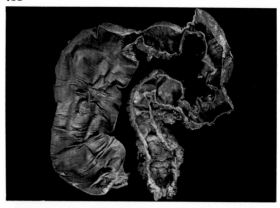

462 **Pseudopolyp from the colon** (4455) of a young man with Crohn's disease who was treated for nine years on steroids and was suffering from faecal fistula. A hemicolectomy with resection of the terminal ileum was carried out and several 'pseudopolyps' were removed from the distal colon. The specimen (left) is a $16 \times 15 \times 6$ mm mass with seven projections on it; these histologically consist of oedematous mucosal folds with dilated lymphatics, intact muscularis mucosa with non-specific chronic inflammatory cell infiltrate in the lamina propria (shown on right). *(H&E × 33)*

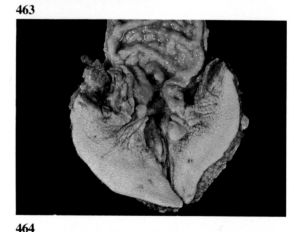

463 **Crohn's disease** (4455) of the anorectal region in a 28-year-old man treated previously by hemicolectomy. Attempted abdominoperineal resection was impossible because of adhesions: 30 cm of the colon and rectum with anus were excised. Close-up shows a serpiginous ulcer (15×15 mm) with undermined edges ramifying for 1 to 2 cm into the anal tissue where there are several anal tags. Sections showed granulomatous ulcerative proctocolitis in keeping with Crohn's disease.

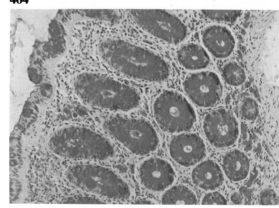

464 **Muciphages in the colonic mucosa** (6951) in a 25-year-old man with Crohn's disease of the terminal ileum but apparently normal large bowel. The section has been stained with Alcian which stains mucin green. The accumulation of muciphages in the lamina propria is seen in colonic mucosa of apparently healthy individuals and is presumably a non-specific manifestation of mucosal injury. *(× 83)*

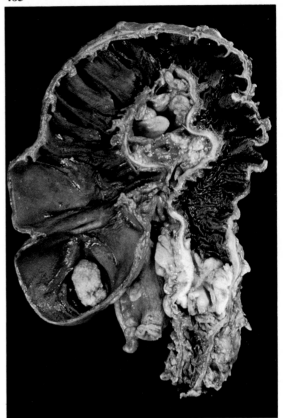

465 Melanosis coli (5711) complicated by two separate adenocarcinomas of the colon, from a 73-year-old woman presenting with subacute intestinal obstruction. The specimen shows black discoloration of the whole 50cm length of the colon and pale neoplasms, one in the caecum and the other 9cm from the cut end of the specimen.

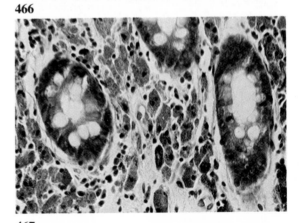

466 Melanosis coli (5711) Section to show pigment-containing macrophages in the lamina propria. *(H&E × 133)*

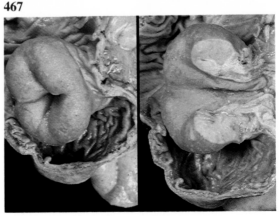

467 Lipomatosis of the ileocaecal valve (7615) from a 76-year-old woman with recurring episodes of subacute obstruction. A hemicolectomy was done: the only remarkable feature was the (3 × 3 × 2 cm) ileocaecal valve (described at the time as looking like a uterine cervix) which shows the typical appearance of pathological adiposity. The orifice was patent. It was felt, in the absence of any other disease, that the lipomatous valve may have been leading to intussusception but at the time of surgery it was still in its normal place. On left the valve intact, on the right after removing a sector for histology which confirmed that the yellow tissue is mature adipose tissue.

468 'Panethoma' of the ascending colon (8140) from a 51-year-old woman with a palpable mass in the right side of the abdomen. Barium enema demonstrated a filling defect. A right hemicolectomy was done: 16 cm from the ileocaecal valve a large (6.5 × 5.5 × 4 cm) cauliflower-like mass fills the lumen. It has a 15 mm wide base into which the muscularis propria is drawn but macroscopically no obvious invasion is seen and no enlarged nodes. Histologically the lesion is a highly cellular papillary adenoma with some areas where Paneth cells predominate – so called panethoma.

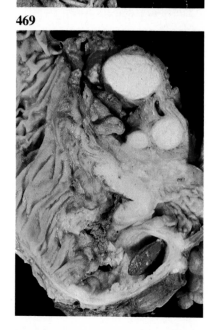

469 Carcinoma of the caecum (8143) with gross lymph node metastases from a 69-year-old woman in whom a barium enema showed a large filling defect. A right hemicolectomy was done: the specimen shows an ulcerated carcinoma (10 cm at its widest) penetrating the muscle coat, infiltrating pericaecal fat and spreading up the colon for 5 cm and into ileocaecal-valve lips. Enlarged nodes (up to 4 cm) are shown in the mesocolon. Histologically the lesion was reported as well-differentiated adenocarcinoma showing extensive lymphatic spread. A prune stone has been held up in the caecum.

470 Carcinoma of the caecum (8143) in a 46-year-old doctor with an 18-month history of progressive tiredness and discovered to have anaemia when using his own blood as a control. On the left photograph shows serosal surface of the caecum just beyond the ileocaecal valve with a dark-red area slightly depressed and with vessels radiating from it. On the right the mucosal surface shows a 3 cm in diameter ulcer with hyperaemic rolled edges 3 cm above the ileocaecal valve on the mesocolonic border where it has penetrated muscle coat and invaded mesocolonic fat for a distance of 1 cm. In the mesocolon adjacent to the neoplasm there are two lymph nodes containing metastases but the nodes proximal to these are free. Three adenomatous polyps are present in the caecum, one opposite the ileocaecal valve, one between the valve and the inferior margin of the carcinoma and the other 8 cm above the ileocaecal valve. Sections were reported as well-differentiated highly cellular (mitoses up to 20 per HP field with abnormal forms) glandular carcinoma with moderate desmoplasia and accompanying round-cell infiltrate: several lymph nodes showed foci of histiocytes and multinucleate giant cells.

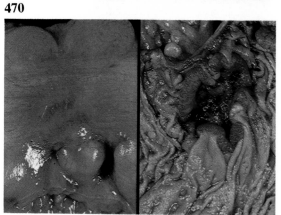

471

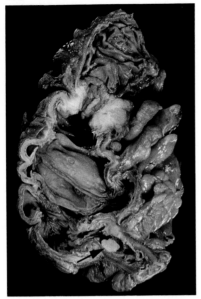

472

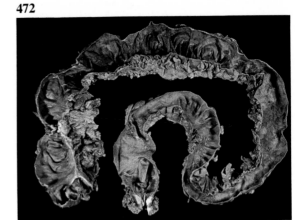

473

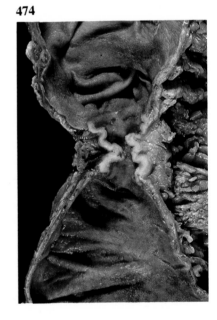

471 Carcinoma of the ascending colon (8143) **with ileal carcinoid** (8243) in a 57-year-old man. The well-differentiated glandular carcinoma forms an annular constriction involving 3.5cm of the wall causing narrowing of the lumen and there is hypertrophy of the muscle coat proximally. The carcinoid tumour (arrowed) (2×1.5cm) shows a yellowish cut surface and penetrates the hypertrophied ileal muscle; carcinoid metastases are present in the nodes in the ileocaecal angle.

472 Carcinoma of the ascending colon (8143) **complicating ulcerative colitis** (4003) of 12 years duration in a 35-year-old man. His symptoms had settled and he was off treatment but on review was found to be anaemic and proctoscopy showed no ulceration. Barium studies indicated a stricture near the hepatic flexure. The specimen consists of the whole colon and rectum with an annular carcinoma (4cm long) situated 9cm distal to the ileocaecal valve. The mucosa varies greatly in appearance – red and thin in the caecum and ascending colon, with sudden transition to darker red and granular mucosa in the transverse colon where there is a stricture, beyond which the rest (30cm) shows ulceration and the dark-red mucosa then changes to pale with linear ulcers forming a lacy pattern, then another stricture. The descending colon shows extensive superficial ulcers separated by granular and atrophic mucosa. The sigmoid is generally narrow and shows linear ulcers and cobblestone mucosa with circumferential ulceration in its distal part and in the upper rectum. The lower rectum is pale and smooth.

474 Carcinoma of the colon (8143) **complicating ulcerative colitis** (4003) Same specimen as in **472** showing the carcinoma in longitudinal section. This patient has only one carcinoma – it is quite common for patients with longstanding chronic ulcerative colitis to develop more than one – we have seen one fatal case with five separate malignant tumours.

473 Carcinoma of the colon (8143) **complicating ulcerative colitis** (4003) Same specimen as in **472** showing the carcinoma as it appears when viewed from either side of the stricture.

474

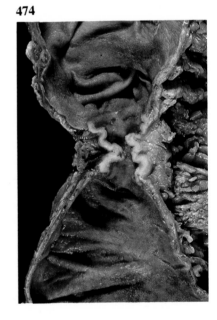

475 Carcinoma of the ascending colon (8143) from a 53-year-old woman who complained of bleeding fresh blood per rectum. Colonoscopy showed an obvious ulcerated tumour, which was excised. It is a highly cellular (mitoses up to 50 per HP field) glandular carcinoma with tubule and acinar formation, showing mucin production and widespread lymphatic permeation and penetrating muscle coat. On the right the section shows hyperchromatic pleomorphic nuclei, some in mitosis, some showing enlarged irregular nucleoli. *(H&E × 133)*

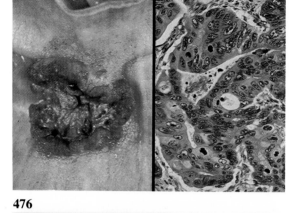

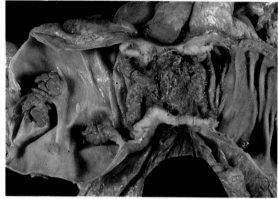

476 Carcinoma of the transverse colon (8143) **with adenomatous polyps** (8210) from a 78-year-old woman with large-bowel obstruction. The 4 cm long annular carcinoma penetrated the muscle coat, but lymph nodes were free of metastases. There are three pedunculated adenomatous polyps distal to the carcinoma: the muscle proximal to it is hypertrophied.

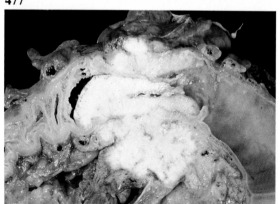

477 Carcinoma of descending colon (8143) (same lesion as in **478**) cut longitudinally to show central 5 cm long annular carcinoma completely replacing the colonic wall and forming a (4 × 3 cm) mass in the mesocolon. Histologically the lesion is partly of solid spheroidal-cell type elsewhere showing glandular differentiation, some areas are necrotic and heavily calcified: dilated lymphatics contain pale staining fluid resembling that seen in the 'cysts' which are of lymphangiectatic type with flat endothelial lining.

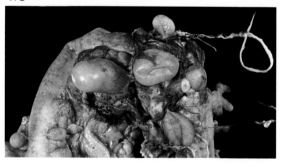

478 Carcinoma of the descending colon (8143) in a 44-year-old woman with abdominal pain and palpable mass. The specimen consists of 35 cm of the colon with its central third the site of multiple cystic polyps (up to 5 cm in diameter) while elongated appendices epiploicae show long 10 to 15 cm string-like tentacles attached to their tip.

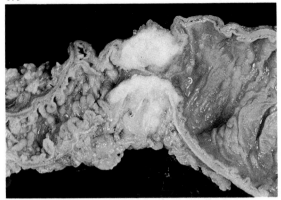

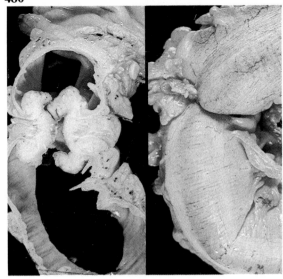

479   Carcinoma of the splenic flexure (8143) in a 40-year-old woman whose mother died of bowel cancer. The 25 cm length of the colon includes a stenosing adenocarcinoma affecting 3.5 cm of the wall reducing the lumen to 4 mm. The mucosa of the colon is studded with innumerable (over 200) adenomatous polyps, up to 10 mm in diameter. The carcinoma penetrated muscle coat but lymph nodes appeared free of metastases.

480   Carcinoma of sigmoid colon (8143) **producing 'string stricture'** in a 75-year-old man admitted with abdominal pain and absolute constipation. The 27 cm of colon included a central carcinomatous stricture, shown in close up on right, and after slicing, on the left. The carcinoma is an annular one and has destroyed 1 to 2 cm of the wall reducing the lumen to a narrow slit.

481

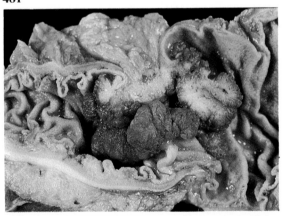

481   Carcinoma of sigmoid colon (8143) forming an exophytic (cauliflower-like) mass 6 cm in diameter in an old woman with calcified fibroids. It is a well-differentiated adenocarcinoma, penetrating the hypertrophied muscle coat but four nodes are uninvolved.

482

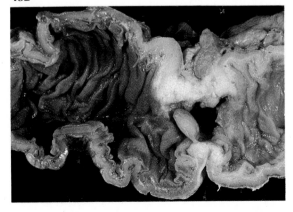

482   Carcinoma of colon (8143) **causing intussusception** in a 52-year-old woman with a history of having had her left ovary removed some months earlier for carcinoma. She had complained of vomiting, pain, abdominal distension and absolute constipation. The carcinoma was annular and ulcerated involving 2.6 cm of the wall. An orange pip was impacted in the base of the ulcer. There was discoloration of the bowel which had intussuscepted.

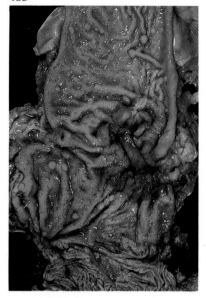

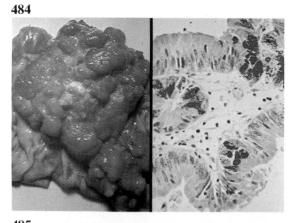

483   Carcinoma of rectum (8143) in a 66-year-old man with a two-month history of passing blood and mucus and a feeling of incomplete emptying of bowel. At rectal examination, a hard ulcerated area was palpable: biopsy showed infiltrating adenocarcinoma. The resected specimen shows the (4 × 3.5 cm) ulcerated carcinoma within 4 cm of the anorectal junction and multiple metaplastic polyps.

484   Carcinoma of rectum (8143) **with abundant Paneth cells:** from a woman who complained of passing blood and mucus and sensation of incomplete defaecation. The 8 cm diameter exophytic carcinoma of the upper rectum was resected. Histologically it shows, on right, a papillary structure where Paneth cells and mucin-secreting columnar cells line the papillary processes. *(Alcian phloxine × 133)*

485   Carcinoma arising in an adenomatous polyp (8143) in a 67-year-old man. The lesion was identified at colonoscopy and segmental resection of upper rectum and sigmoid carried out. The neoplastic mass (7 × 5 cm) showed at one end a villous papillomatous appearance and at the other a solid papillomatous appearance, while centrally adjacent to an indrawn area of serosa and mesocolon there is a hard mucoid 2 cm area of infiltrating carcinoma. Histologically the pattern ranged from benign adenoma (showing an unusually large complement of Paneth cells) through highly cellular papillary adenoma to infiltrating adenocarcinoma with mucoid areas.

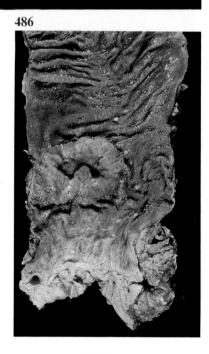

486   Carcinoma of rectum (8143) in a 71-year-old woman with history of taking purgatives 'all her life'. The unpigmented 4.5 × 3.5 cm ulcerated carcinoma and metaplastic polyps are conspicuous against the almost black mucosa caused by melanosis.

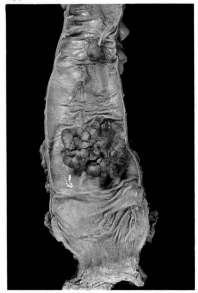

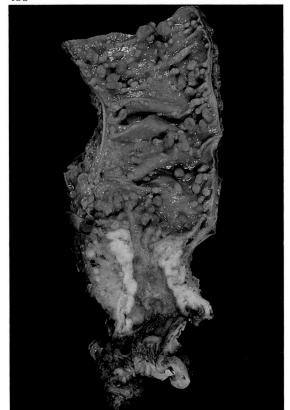

487 Carcinoma of rectum (8143) with adenomatous polyp in sigmoid colon in a 62-year-old man who complained of altered bowel habit and passing blood per rectum. The specimen shows, 10cm above the anorectal junction an 8×6cm exophytic carcinoma affecting all but 4cm of the circumference. A pedunculated adenomatous polyp measures 15×15mm on a 3.5cm stalk. Two smaller polyps were proximal to the large one.

488 Carcinoma of rectum (8143) **complicating polyposis coli** (8220) in a 32-year-old woman who complained of chronic perianal sepsis. At laparotomy a tumour was found and removed by abdominoperineal excision including the invaded vaginal wall. The specimen comprises 24cm of sigmoid colon and rectum with an 8cm long ulcerated annular carcinoma reaching to within 2.5cm of the anorectal junction. The mucosa is studded with adenomatous polyps (up to 1.5cm).

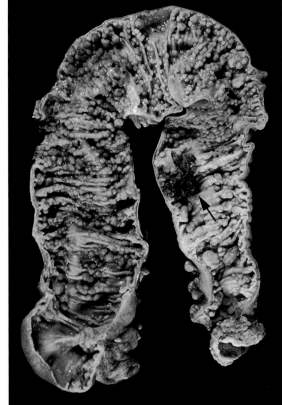

489 Polyposis coli (8220) Remainder of the colon removed from a patient whose rectum is shown in **488**. There are innumerable adenomatous polyps including a quite large (4×3.5cm) one (arrowed) which histologically appeared highly cellular.

490 Villous papilloma of rectum (8261) from a 60-year-old woman who had a hysterectomy and developed hypopotassaemia: on sigmoidoscopy an 8cm long villous papillary lesion was seen encircling the upper rectum. A pull-through technique was used to resect the affected area along with 20cm of the colon. Histologically the lesion was benign and showed abundant mucin-secreting columnar cells and patches where Paneth cells and Kulchitsky cells were also present.

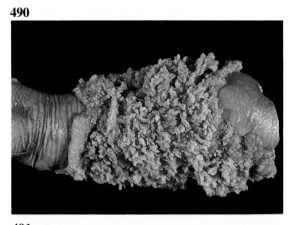

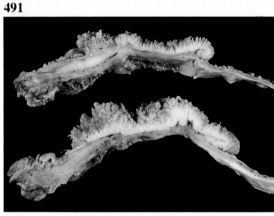

491 Villous papilloma of rectum (carpet lesion) (8261) Another example with the 6cm long circumferential lesion extending down to the anorectal junction and treated by abdominoperineal resection. The patient was a 74-year-old man with an 18-month history of frequent mucous diarrhoea and severe electrolyte imbalance.

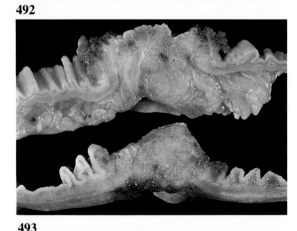

492 Mucoid carcinoma of colon (8483) in a 53-year-old doctor who complained of rectal bleeding. A 4cm diameter ulcerated carcinoma involves all but 1.5cm of the circumference of the bowel. The margin is red, in places papillary, but the bulk of the lesion is solid and mucoid. Three nodes close to the tumour are replaced by metastases, but four others near the plane of excision were free. Serosal tissue over the carcinoma show mucoid carcinoma infiltrating very close to the surface which showed fibrinous peritonitis.

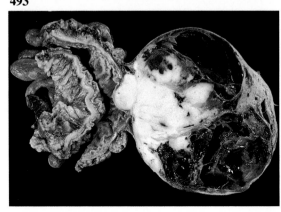

493 Leiomyosarcoma of colon (8893) from a 51-year-old woman with abdominal swelling, thought to be caused by an ovarian cyst but at laparotomy was found to have a 12cm diameter spherical tumour arising from the wall of the pelvic colon. Histologically it was reported as a leiomyosarcoma, with electronmicrographic evidence that the spindle cells showed longitudinal fibrillary component and transverse banding. The 10cm length of opened colon is shown with the spherical mass arising from the muscularis propria. The cut surface is partly pale pink with solid areas, and partly haemorrhagic and necrotic with cystic areas; the mucosa overlying it appears intact, and there were no metastases.

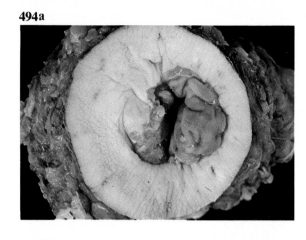

494a

494a Carcinomatous recurrence in colostomy (8013) two years after abdominoperineal resection for carcinoma of rectum in a 64-year-old man. The specimen is a 5 cm circular piece of skin with hard nodular inferior margin to the colostomy.

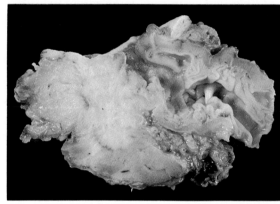

494b

494b Carcinomatous recurrence in colostomy (8013) Lesion sliced to show a mass (3.5cm) of infiltrating carcinomatous tissue extending deeply to within less than 5mm of the plane of resection.

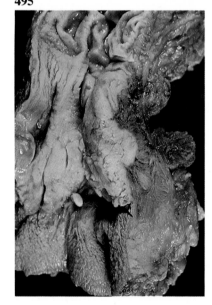

495

495 Basaloid type of squamous-cell carcinoma (8123) of the anus from a 70-year-old dancing teacher with a history of bleeding per rectum for six months and who had complained of something protruding from the anus. An abdominoperineal resection was done: the plaque-like tumour mass (4 × 3 cm) involves the whole length of the anal canal and protrudes into the rectum. Histologically the lesion was predominantly of well-differentiated basaloid type, superficially invasive in that muscle coats are not infiltrated.

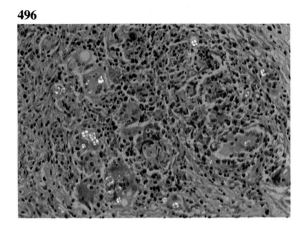

496 Starch granuloma (4410) in the form of a nodule on the surface of the intestine of a 49-year-old woman who complained of pain in the RIF. She had been operated on one month earlier for duodenal ulcer. An appendicectomy and division of adhesions was done. The serosa of the appendix, adhesions and omentum and the mesenteric nodule all showed starch granuloma. Section viewed, with partial polarised light, shows birefringent starch grains in macrophages among granulation tissue infiltrated by eosinophil polymorphonuclear leucocytes, some lymphocytes plasma cells and histiocytes. *(H&E × 53: partly polarised)*

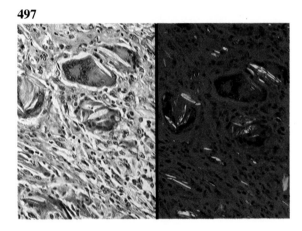

497 Talc granuloma (4410) from the umbilicus of a four-month-old baby girl: the mother was concerned about a pink-red pedunculated (1.2 cm) mass projecting from the umbilicus. Sections show granulomatous inflammation with talc crystals mainly in phagocytes, including multinucleate giant cells. On the right the section is shown viewed with polarised light and a first order red compensator. Final proof of its being talc was obtained by incinerating a duplicate section at 650°C. The birefringent crystals were unchanged. *(H&E × 83)*

7 Urinary tract and male genitalia

Kidney (T72)

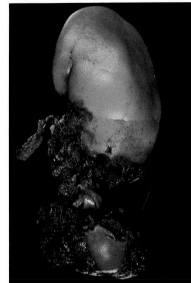

498

498 Ruptured left kidney (1803) from a seven-year-old girl who was involved in road traffic accident. The kidney was received in two parts, one piece (7×4×3cm) includes the pelvis and a haematoma at the lower pole and the other piece (5×3cm) is embedded in a clot. Histologically there was *no* significant abnormality other than that caused by trauma. The lacerated spleen (30g) was also removed.

499 Calcium oxalate urinary stones (3100) A selection showing the range of size, shape and colour: they are either honey-coloured if 'pure' crystalline (dihydrate) or light to dark-brown (altered blood), quite hard and usually radio-opaque and show concentric laminae and radial striae resembling mulberry, or jackstone (2cm) or primula head. Combined with phosphate (usually white to cream colour) they may form a nucleus or darker layers of mixed laminated calculus.

499

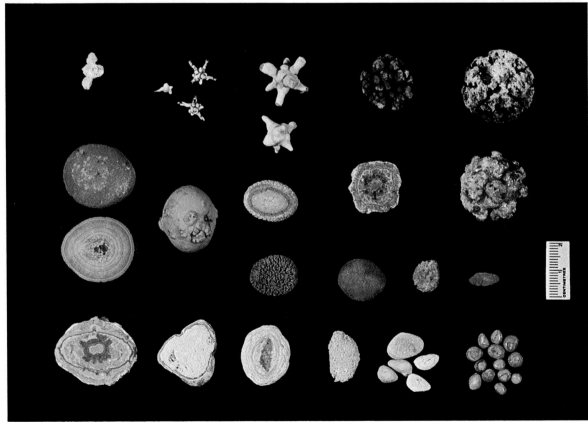

500a Calcium oxalate stones (3100) Small (1 mm to 2 mm) 'pearly' facetted, often tetrahedral calculi.

500b Calcium oxalate stones (3100) Two irregular spiky calculi removed from the prostate bed.

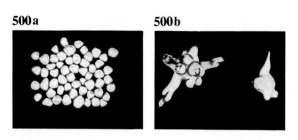

500a 500b

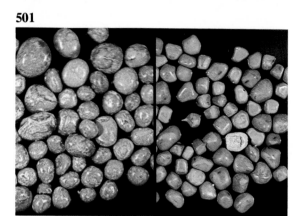

501

501 Calcium oxalate stones (3100) On the left a small 2 mm to 5 mm 'pebble-like' calculi; on the right small (2 mm to 3 mm) 'hemp-seed'-like calculi with tiny spines.

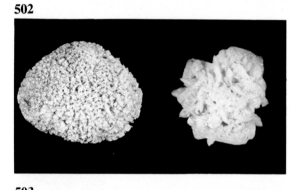

502

502 Calcium oxalate stones (3100) Two examples of large (1.5 cm to 2 cm) honey-coloured spiky calcium oxalate dihydrate calculi. These tend to occur in non-infected urinary tract whereas the laminated and mulberry-like stones with radial striae are found in patients with urinary tract infection.

503

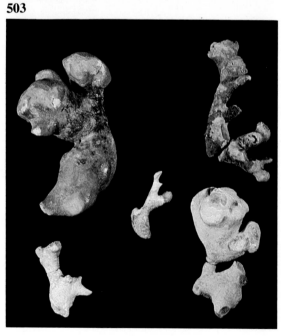

503 Calcium phosphate renal stones (3101) Five examples of staghorn calculi, the shape being a perfect cast of the pelvicalyceal system. These usually contain both carbonate apatite and infective triple phosphate. The smallest is 3 cm long, the largest 10 cm long.

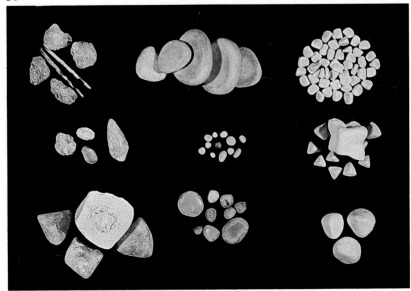

504 Calcium phosphate bladder stone (multiple)
(3101) from nine different patients, to show the general
white to cream colour, the varied shape (5mm) round
to oval, cubes up to 2.5cm, tetrahedrons, and large
3cm discs, and irregular 1cm lumps accompanying an
encrusted hairgrip.

505

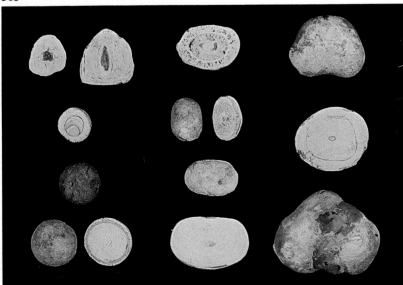

505 Calcium phosphate bladder stone (3101) Twelve
examples of solitary vesical stones. They are either
spherical, ovoid or roughly the shape of the lumen of
the bladder. Generally white and laminated sometimes
with a nucleus of calcium oxalate or foreign material.

506

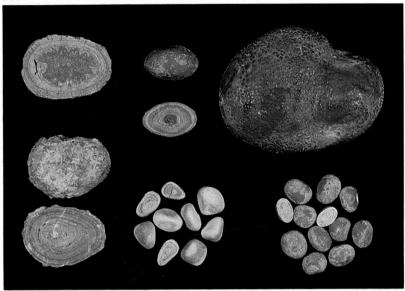

506 **Urate and uric-acid stones** (3103) from the urinary bladder – eight examples. The smallest ones (1 cm) are facetted and light to dark brown. The very large one is 10 cm in diameter and has a Morocco-leather-like surface. On cutting these stones with a lapidary saw one sees beautiful agate-like structure. Any disease leading to hyperuricaemia is liable to be associated with urate/uric-acid stones.

507

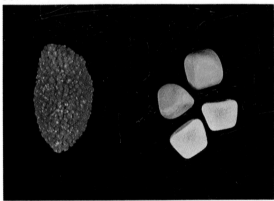

507 **Cystine stones** (3105) from two patients suffering from cystinuria; the urine may show cystine crystals (hexagons) and on chromatography will show excess cystine, lysine and arginine.

508

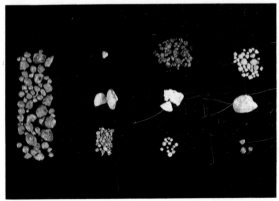

508 **Prostatic calculi** (3106) Examples from 10 patients. They are a mixture of calcium phosphate and calcium oxalate and are most commonly found in enlarged prostatic glands. They are generally very small (1 mm to 2 mm) but can be up to 1 cm.

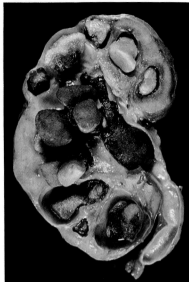

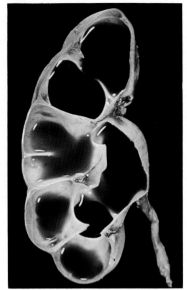

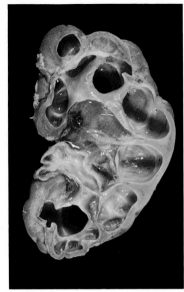

509 Chronic pyelonephritis (4302) **and hydronephrosis with staghorn calculus** (3101) from a 51-year-old woman with a long history of recurrent urinary-tract infection, a mass in the right hypochondrium and a large staghorn calculus visible on xray in the right kidney. The dilated pelvis (4 × 3 cm) is filled with calculus and the cortex is paper thin in places. There were two stenoses in the proximal ureter which is dilated.

510 Hydronephrosis of right kidney (3520) in a five-year-old girl with sudden onset of frank haematuria and vomiting for one day and no previous history of kidney trouble. The specimen is an enlarged (17 × 10 cm) right kidney with a ragged tear in the posterior wall of the upper calyx. All the calyces are dilated and filled with brown fluid. The section showed hydronephrotic atrophy, and chronic inflammation of the lining of the pelvis and calyces. The appearances were regarded as having followed trauma to the child's back ('battered' child).

511 Hydronephrosis of right kidney (3520) in a 15-year-old boy with a history of ten episodes of renal colic in the space of three years and increased frequency of micturition (10 × day; 1 × night). IVP showed non-functioning right kidney. The kidney measures 10.5 × 6.5 cm and the dilated pelvicalyceal system is full of clear urine. The cortex and medulla are thinned to less than 5 mm in thickness. No aberrant vessels were identified. The upper 4 cm of the ureter was not dilated and the cause of the hydronephrosis was not established.

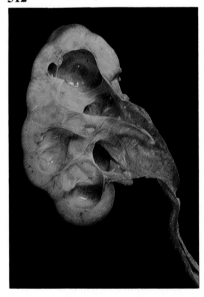

512 Hydronephrosis of right kidney (3520) in a 55-year-old foreman joiner who first noted haematuria four months earlier when cystoscopy showed NAD. IVP revealed a non-functioning right kidney and his blood pressure was 180/120 mm Hg. Retrograde pyelogram showed an obstruction at the lower end of the ureter and this proved to be a transitional cell carcinoma (see **535**). The kidney (9 × 5 × 4 cm) shows reduction of parenchyma to 1 cm, and dilatation of pelvis and all calyces.

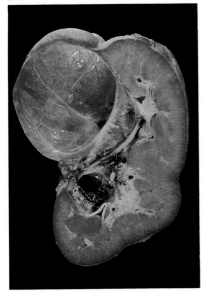

513 **Solitary cyst of left kidney** (3540)
in a 63-year-old man who complained
of haematuria. Radiological studies
showed a large cyst at the upper pole.
The kidney is $12 \times 7 \times 6$ cm with 7 cm
thin-walled unilocular cyst filled with
clear fluid and lined by a single layer
of flattened epithelial cells. The only
other remarkable feature histologically was severe arteriosclerosis
and prominent juxtaglomerular
apparatus.

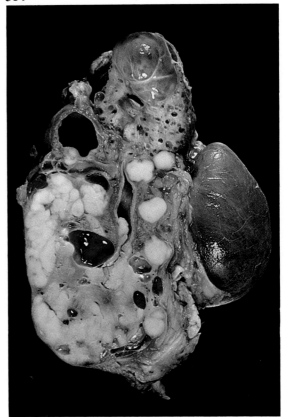

514 **Polycystic disease of kidneys** (3558) **complicated
by carcinoma** (8313), from a 72-year-old man known to
have polycystic kidneys and who complained of loin
pain and haematuria. At operation malignant neoplasm
in the single kidney was seen to be invading the vena
cava. The kidney is bulky (weight 850 g – 19.5×10
$\times 7$ cm) and polycystic: cysts up to 9 cm in diameter
replace most of the parenchyma and at one pole there is
a solid bosselated firm neoplasm infiltrating between
cysts through capsule, into pelvis and veins. Histolo-
logically it is a very varied renal carcinoma ranging
from papillary columnar cell to undifferentiated
spheroidal cell, with some desmoplasia and sparse
lymphocytic infiltrate.

515

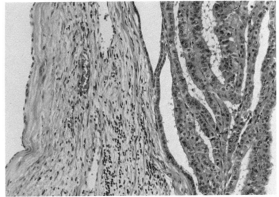

515 **Polycystic disease of kidneys** (3558) **complicated
by renal carcinoma** (8313): section of lesion shown in
514. Simple cyst wall is seen on the left while on the
right there is trabecular arrangement of proliferating
cuboidal and columnar cells mainly with eosinophilic
granular cytoplasm. *(H&E × 53)*

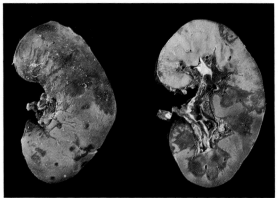

516

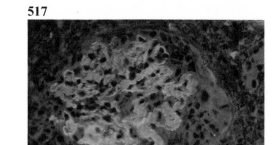

517

516 Infarcts (5740) **and haemorrhages** (3850) **in kidney** of an 11-year-old girl hit in the back in a road traffic accident. She had a large left retroperitoneal haematoma and the left kidney (120 g; 10 × 7 × 4 cm) shows a dark-red mottled outer surface; a ragged stump of renal artery and vein was recognisable alongside the pelvis which was full of blood clot. The cut surface shows infarction of nearly one half of the kidney and smaller areas of cortical necrosis.

517 Rapidly progressive proliferative glomerulo-nephritis (4001) Renal biopsy from 65-year-old woman with proteinuria, haematuria and raised ESR. This preparation demonstrates the presence of IgG as bright apple-green linear staining of the basement membrane by an immunofluorescent technique using an FITC conjugate. The background and crescent show red fluorescence from counterstaining. Electronmicroscopy showed diffuse thickening of basement membranes with few small electron-dense lumps in and around the basement membrane, in keeping with antiglomerular basement membrane glomerulonephritis. *(× 83)*

518 Xanthogranulomatous pyelonephritis (4402) in a 59-year-old woman with left renal pain and recurrent UTI, known hypertensive and losing weight. IVP showed non-functioning left kidney. It was enlarged (14 × 8 × 6 cm; weight 440 g). The pelvis is filled with green pus with calcified material in it. The parenchyma is reduced to 1 cm in many places, and the capsule is adherent. Histologically the appearances were those of xanthogranulomatous pyelonephritis. No AAFB were seen and Mycobacteria were not isolated.

518

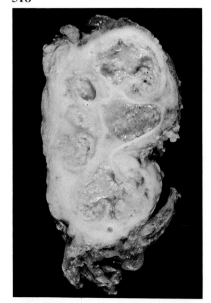

519

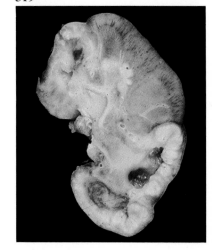

519 Xanthogranulomatous pyelonephritis (4402) in a 24-year-old woman who had a perinephric abscess that burst into the colon – this was treated by nephrostomy and hemicolectomy, then an elective nephrectomy. The kidney weighs 100 g and is 10 × 6 × 4 cm. The cut surface shows dilated calyces with renal parenchyma replaced by yellow solid masses, which on histological examination proved to consist of masses of lipid-containing macrophages in granulation tissue. This is a good example of an appearance where confusion with neoplasm or tuberculosis could easily arise.

520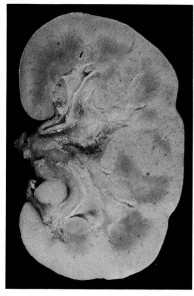

521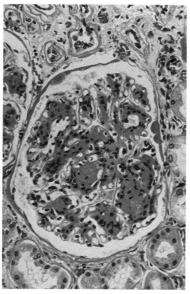

522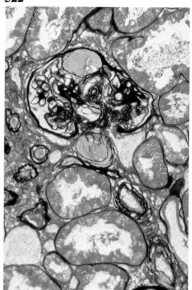

520 Diabetic kidney (5332) with granulomatous ureteritis from a 49-year-old man with a six-month history of haematuria and left loin pain. Xray showed intramural tumour at lower end of left ureter – this proved to be a granulomatous ureteritis and periureteritis of uncertain aetiology. The sections of kidney, which was large and pale (18 × 11 × 8 cm), showed unusually severe hyaline arteriolosclerosis and irregular thickening of the peritubular basement membranes, in keeping with long-standing diabetes mellitus with hypertension.

521 Diabetic glomerulosclerosis (5332) Glomerulus showing Kimmelstiel-Wilson nodular glomerulosclerosis and lozenges on Bowman's capsule. *(H&E × 83)*

522 Diabetic glomerulosclerosis (5332) and hyaline arterioles: section stained with PACAMS toned with gold chloride. The hyaline in the arteriole and on Bowman's capsule is rose pink: the basement membrane is black and that around atrophic tubules is wrinkled and thickened. *(PACAMS × 53)*

523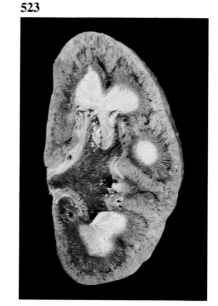

524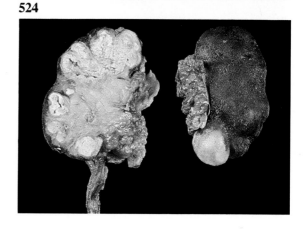

523 Papillary necrosis (necrotising papillitis) (5455) caused by phenacetin abuse: there is also a severe haemorrhagic pyelitis.

524 Tuberculosis of the kidney and ureter (4470) in a 48-year-old man who complained of loin pain and on xray showed contracted calcified non-functioning right kidney. The specimen (7 × 3 × 2.5 cm) with 7.5 cm of thickened ureter weighs 60 g. The outer surface appears lobulated, one dilated calyx appearing white at one pole. The cut surface shows caseous material replacing nearly all of the parenchyma and areas of calcification. Sections confirmed the diagnosis of tuberculous pyelo-uretero-nephritis. Culture of caseous material grew Mycobacterium tuberculosis.

525

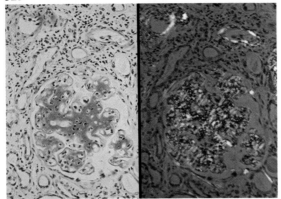

526

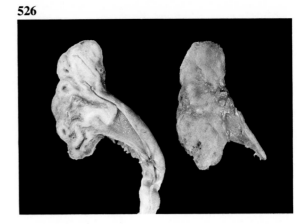

525 Amyloid disease in the kidney (5510) from a 71-year-old man with a history of pulmonary tuberculosis and diagnosis of amyloidosis established on rectal mucosa biopsy. This section on left shows a glomerulus and arteriole stained with congo red and on right when viewed with polarising microscope exhibits dichroic birefringence. *(Congo red × 53)*

526 Hypoplasia of left kidney (7030) from an eight-year-old boy with a non-functioning left kidney. It is small (4 × 2 × 1.3 cm) with thick-walled pelvis and ureter. Histologically only a few immature-looking glomeruli were seen, most of the medulla was fibrous and there were severe chronic inflammatory changes in the wall of the pelvis and the ureter.

527

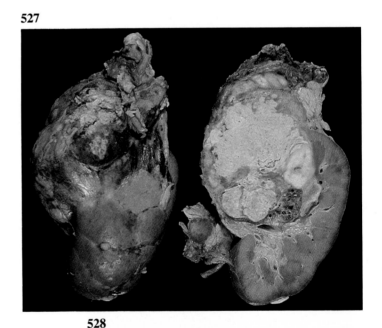

527 Renal carcinoma (hypernephroma) (8313) of the left kidney from a 57-year-old man with pyrexia, and a mass in the left loin. The specimen is an enlarged kidney (13 × 6 × 5 cm) with upper pole replaced by a large (9 cm) neoplasm, part of which projects into the upper calyx as a (3 × 1.2 cm) white tongue. The neoplasm penetrates the capsule and invades the attached adrenal gland. At the lower pole a 2 cm spherical metastasis lies in a lymph node in fat in front of the ureter. Sections showed clear-cell carcinoma arranged in trabeculae and alveoli but with spindle-cell pattern in places.

528

528 Renal carcinoma (8313) Section to show clear-cell pattern in paraffin section. The clearness results from the loss of cytoplasmic lipid and glycogen during paraffin processing: on the left the clear-cell carcinoma is seen to have penetrated the wall of a vein and is growing within its lumen. *(H&E × 53 × 133)*

529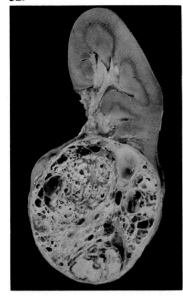

530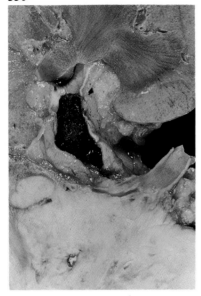

531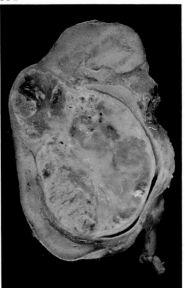

529 Renal carcinoma (8313) at lower pole of left kidney from woman with palpable mass in the left loin. The spherical (7cm in diameter) neoplasm shows the typical variegated colour on the cut surface – the red areas of haemorrhage, the yellow-orange lipid-rich neoplasm and the greyish areas of stroma. The capsule of this clear-cell carcinoma showed multiple foci of calcification: there are cysts of varied size throughout the tumour.

530 Renal carcinoma (8313) from 53-year-old man with anaemia and haematuria for four weeks. A tumour was identified on xray at the lower pole and nephrectomy carried out. A 10cm diameter firm mass of yellowish white colour extended to the renal capsule and penetrated it in four places. There was infiltration into the upper calyx with haemorrhage; the calyx and pelvis being filled with blood clot is shown in closeup.

531 Renal carcinoma (8313) from a 49-year-old woman with mass in the right loin and non-functioning right kidney. The enlarged kidney (15 × 12 × 9 cm) has its central part replaced by a lobulated carcinoma, which has pushed the lateral pelvic wall medially compressing the pelvis into a narrow slit. The cut surface shows typical red, yellow and grey colour.

532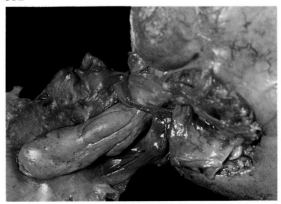

532 Carcinoma of kidney (8313) invading renal veins and inferior vena cava.

157

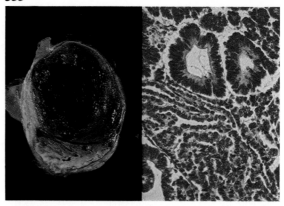

533 Wilm's tumour (nephroblastoma) (8963) removed at heminephrectomy from a seven-year-old boy with bilateral renal tumours. The specimen is a 7 cm diameter mass with a (4.5 × 3.5 × 3 cm) part of the left kidney, together weighing 108 g. The cut surface of the mass is largely haemorrhagic with only a narrow pale area towards one side. Histologically the section shows typical appearance of nephroblastoma. *(H&E × 83)*

534

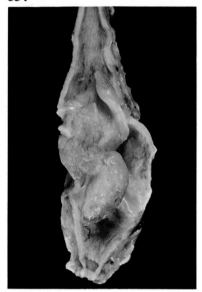

Ureter (T73)

534 Ureteric polyp (8120) from a 73-year-old woman with one episode of haematuria and found to have left ureteric obstruction and non-functioning hydronephrotic left kidney. The tumour consists of a thin (1.2 × 0.5 cm) polyp projecting upwards and a thick (2.5 × 1.2 × 1 cm) polyp hanging down with a sessile (1.5 × 1 × 1 cm) mass between them; histologically the lesion was mainly transitional cell papilloma but showed nuclear pleomorphism and aberrant mitoses which warranted a diagnosis of carcinoma.

535

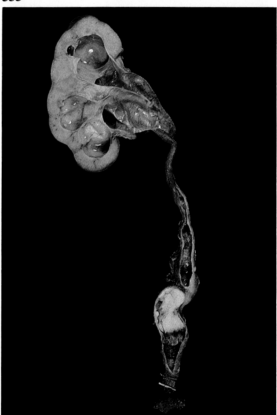

535 Transitional-cell carcinoma of ureter (8123) Lesion causing obstruction and hydronephrosis shown in **512**. The ureter is dilated (2 cm in diameter) in its lower part where a large papillary and solid neoplasm involves a 4 cm length of the wall and plugs the lumen. Histologically it is a transitional-cell carcinoma, highly cellular (mitoses up to 10 per HP field with abnormal forms) and more solid than papillary. Invasion appeared confined to the lamina propria. Multiple foci of papillary transitional neoplastic change of similar appearance to the main lesion were present along the length of the ureter, but the pelvis was free of neoplasm.

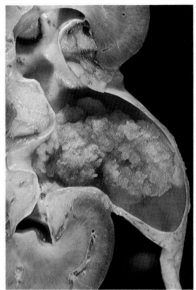

536

536 Transitional-cell carcinoma of the pelvis (8123) of the left kidney from a 38-year-old man who complained of intermittent haematuria for six months. IVP showed a filling defect in the left renal pelvis. Close-up shows (4×2.5 cm) solid and papillary lesion involving the anterior wall of the pelvis. It is a transitional-cell carcinoma, moderately cellular (mitoses up to 6 per HP field) and invades but does not penetrate the muscle coat. Sections of the 10 cm of ureter resected with the kidney showed no other lesions.

Bladder (T74)

537

537 Ectopia vesicae (2510) from a three-year-old girl. The specimen is the excised bladder with distal ends of both ureters. It is a (6×6 cm) mass with intensely congested, oedematous, chronically inflamed, partly ulcerated mucosa which is continuous at the margin with skin. Histologically the mucosal pattern varied greatly, in places covered by transitional-cell epithelium, elsewhere showing mucin-secreting columnar epithelium. No evidence of malignancy was seen. The final report was ectopia vesicae with chronic cystitis and glandular metaplasia. *(H&E × 13)*

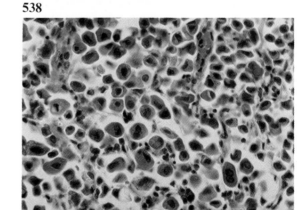

538

538 Malakoplakia of the urinary bladder (4555) from a 61-year-old woman. Section shows characteristic large mononuclear-cell infiltrate of the bladder wall and intracytoplasmic globular inclusions (Michaelis–Gutman bodies). *(H&E × 133)*

539

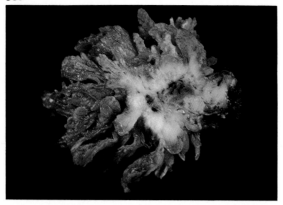

539 Transitional-cell papilloma of the urinary bladder (8120), from a 47-year-old woman with a history of repeated attacks of haematuria for three years. The specimen is a papillary mass ($5 \times 3 \times 3$ cm) on a (1.5×1 cm) base.

540

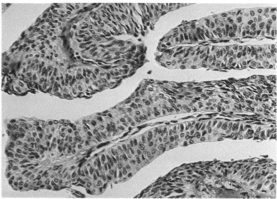

540 Transitional-cell papilloma of the urinary bladder (8120) Section shows papillary processes covered by four to nine layers of transitional-cell epithelium. There is little nuclear pleomorphism, mitoses were scanty; no evidence of invasion of the bladder wall at the base of the lesion was seen. *(H&E × 83)*

541

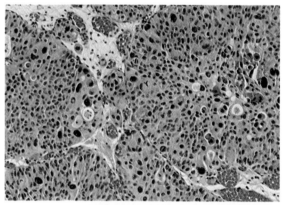

541 Transitional-cell carcinoma of the urinary bladder (8123) from a 47-year-old man with tumours recurring at short intervals (months) and under treatment with instillation of cytotoxic drugs. Section shows transitional-cell carcinoma with pleomorphic nuclei and mitotic activity including abnormal forms. *(H&E × 83)*

542

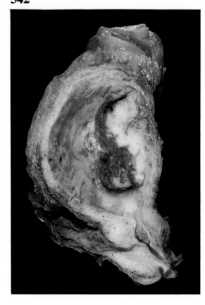

542 Carcinoma of the bladder (8123) from a 50-year-old man. The specimen consists of urinary bladder ($10 \times 10 \times 8$ cm) with trabeculated wall and enlarged prostate gland. The anterior wall of the bladder is the site of a sessile ($5 \times 4 \times 3$ cm) neoplastic mass with ulcerated reddened surface. The cut surface is pale and the carcinoma (well-differentiated transitional-cell type) penetrates the muscle coat. The prostate gland shows moderate benign enlargement.

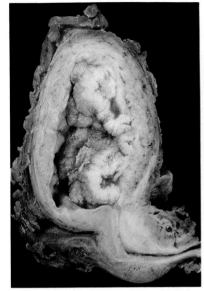

543   **543 Carcinoma of the bladder** (8123) from a 55-year-old labourer with recurrent carcinoma. The specimen is a complete urinary bladder (10×9×7cm) with enlarged prostate gland (5×4×4cm) and 15cm of urethra. The mucosa of the anterior and lateral walls of the bladder is replaced by papillary and solid transitional-cell carcinoma which invades muscle for only a very short distance. No lesions were seen in many sections of the urethral mucosa.

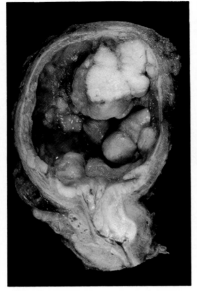

544   **544 Carcinoma of the bladder** (8123) from a 66-year-old man who complained of intermittent haematuria; radiographs showed filling defect. The specimen is a complete urinary bladder (8×8×8cm) with enlarged prostate gland (5×4×4cm). The bladder carcinoma affects all but the upper posterior part of the wall, forming masses up to 3cm in thickness. Histologically it was a poorly differentiated transitional-cell carcinoma permeating lymphatics in the wall, showing only limited invasion of bladder wall though infiltrating the anterior lobe of the prostate gland.

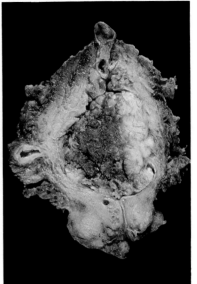

545   **545 Carcinoma of the bladder** (8123) from a 68-year-old man with a history of prostatism. The bladder (10×8×5cm) lumen is filled by papillary and solid neoplasm affecting all but the right upper wall. There is considerable oedema of the mucosa: the muscle coat is hypertrophied and there are two diverticula. The prostate gland shows appearances of benign glandulocystic fibromuscular hyperplasia. Histologically the bladder carcinoma is of well-differentiated transitional-cell type and appears not to invade muscle coat.

546 Carcinoma of the bladder (8123) treated by radiotherapy, followed four weeks later by radical cystectomy with hysterectomy and bilateral salpingo-oöphorectomy in a 59-year-old woman in whom a poorly differentiated transitional-cell carcinoma of the bladder was diagnosed on biopsy. The specimen shows urinary bladder, urethra and uterus with multiple fibroids. The bladder is contracted and its wall shows oedematous nodules over an area (4×4cm) on the postero-inferior wall with smaller areas superiorly. A small (5mm) sessile smooth nodule lies at the fundus. Sections showed post-radiation changes and probably variable transitional-cell carcinoma in lymphatics in the lamina propria. The fat on the superolateral aspect of the bladder appeared yellow and opaque as a result of fat necrosis. Nodes from common iliac, external iliac and obturator sites showed no metastases.

546

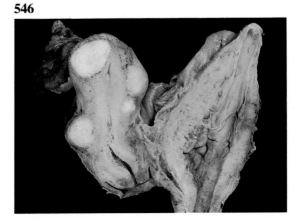

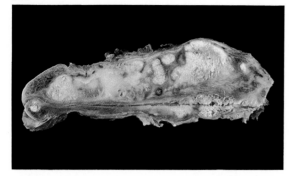

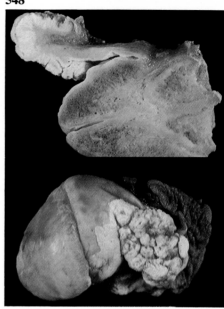

Penis (T76)

547   Metastatic transitional-cell carcinoma in the penis (8016) of a 51-year-old fishmonger who had a cystectomy for carcinoma 10 months earlier after having had repeated cystoscopic treatments for transitional-cell neoplasm for six years. The penile involvement became apparent four months after cystectomy was treated by radiotherapy without much effect and so amputation was done. The specimen is an amputated penis 17cm long with ulcerated lesion on the glans; multiple pale necrotic metastases replace much of the corpora cavernosa, spongiosa, and urethral mucosa posteriorly.

548   Squamous-cell papillary carcinoma of the prepuce (8073) from a 54-year-old engineer. The cauliflower-like mass (2.5 × 1.5cm) occupied an area of prepuce showing pale altered mucosa which histologically showed appearances of intraepithelial (in situ) squamous-cell carcinoma.

549

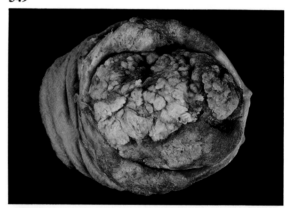

549   Squamous-cell carcinoma of the glans penis (8073) from a 69-year-old man. The lesion involved about two-thirds of the glans and the prepuce which shows red roughened areas. Histologically the white warty parts are well-differentiated squamous-cell carcinoma. There are widespread intraepithelial (in situ) carcinomatous foci on both glans and prepuce and severe chronic inflammation.

550

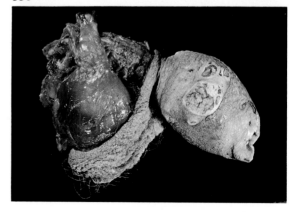

550   Carcinoma of the glans penis ulcerating through the prepuce (8073) of a 64-year-old hackle setter. The lesion was a keratinising squamous-cell carcinoma involving 3.5cm of glans and infiltrating it to a depth of 1.5cm.

551

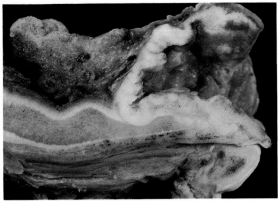

552

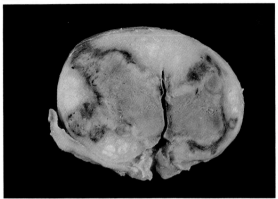

551 Squamous-cell carcinoma of the penis (8073) in a 70-year-old man. The lesion (4.3 cm in length), histologically a squamous-cell carcinoma, has destroyed nearly all of the glans, yet the patient maintained that it had only started three months earlier.

Prostate gland (T77)

552 Infarcts of the prostate gland (5470) from a 68-year-old man with acute urinary retention after a hip replacement operation. The enlarged (5 × 4 × 4 cm) gland weighed 43 g and the cut surface shows a yellow-brown periurethral zone with surrounding dark red-brown periphery. Sections confirmed the clinical diagnosis of benign prostate enlargement (glandulocystic fibromuscular hyperplasia) with recent infarction and prominent squamous metaplasia at the periphery.

553 Prostatic enlargement (glandulocystic fibromuscular hyperplasia) (7300) in a 75-year-old man admitted with acute retention of urine after a long history of prostatism. The enlarged lateral lobes of (6 × 5 × 4 cm) prostate gland weigh 145 g and show nodular hyperplasia of both fibromuscular stroma and glandular elements with cyst formation. The cut surface is pink to light brown and a milky fluid exudes from transected nodules. Carcinoma does not occur commonly in such a gland but when it does, it is usually recognisable by its firmer consistency and yellow-grey colour.

553

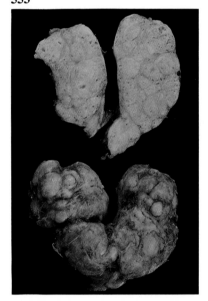

554

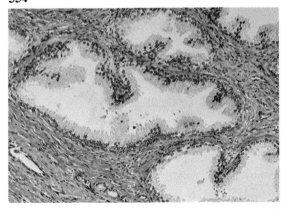

554 Prostate enlargement (7300) Section of a gland shown in **553**. Acini lined by tall, clear epithelial cells forming papillary projections into the dilated lumens are separated by hyperplastic fibromuscular stroma. In very large glands there is usually round-cell (both lymphocytes and plasma cells) infiltration of stroma as well as acute inflammatory foci with neutrophil polymorphonuclear leucocytes: small calculi often form in dilated acini and ducts. *(H&E × 53)*

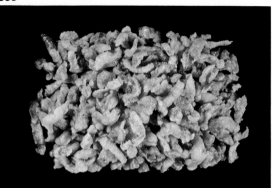

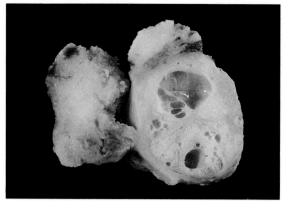

555 **Prostatic enlargement** (7300) Chips of prostatic tissue weighing 120g removed from an 86-year-old retired journalist with prostatism. None of the pieces show the yellow cast and hardness of carcinoma: representative sections showed no evidence of malignancy.

556 **Metastatic transitional-cell carcinoma** (8016) in

the enlarged prostate gland of a 79-year-old man known to have carcinoma of the bladder. The specimen is an irregular mass (4.5×3.5cm) of prostate tissue showing large cysts and nodular hyperplasia with pale friable neoplasm in places papillary. Sections were examined by histochemical method for acid phosphatase with negative results corroborating the diagnosis of metastatic bladder carcinoma.

557

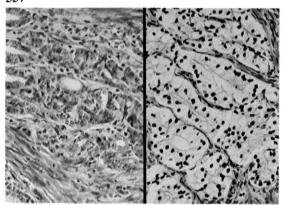

557 **Carcinoma of the prostate gland** (8143) on the left before and on the right after a year's treatment with oestrogen, showing characteristic clear balloon-cell pattern and densely staining nuclei. (H&E×83)

558

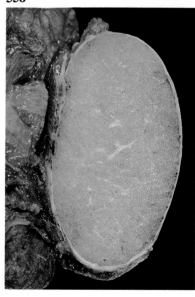

Testis (T78)

558 **Cryptorchid testis** (2314) from a 26-year-old man who complained of a swelling in the inguinal region. A (4×2.5×2cm) testis with uniform brown cut surface and showing no spermatogenesis and without any tumour. The risk of cryptorchid developing a neoplasm is said to be increased 35 times compared with the normal.

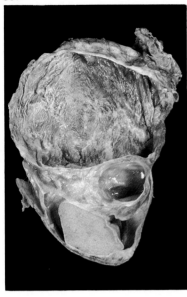

559

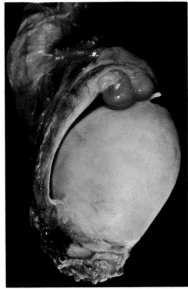

560

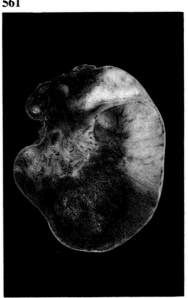

561

559 Hydrocoele of the cord (3532), **epididymal cyst** (3540) **and atrophic testis** (7100) from a 65-year-old man with a 10-year history of a swelling in the groin. It had been drained on several occasions but kept recurring. The hydrocoele is 7.5cm in diameter, the epididymal cyst 2cm in diameter. Accumulation of fluid in the tunica vaginalis forms a pear-shaped swelling in the scrotum. No obvious cause may be found but a search for disease of testis, epididymis or lymphatics is necessary. The specimen shows typical appearance of the lining of a chronic hydrocoele, the whitish areas are fibrous plaques resulting from organised exudate. Histologically it is lined by flattened squames and cuboidal cells.

560 Epididymal cyst (3540) from a 78-year-old man with recurrent inguinal hernia: the right testis was removed at time of repair. Specimen shows two small (10mm and 7mm) cysts at the upper pole of the epididymis: they may be of developmental origin or caused by obstruction of the ducts: those which contain spermatozoa show turbid contents and are more correctly called 'spermatocoele'. Diagnosis is best achieved by aspirating some of the fluid and examining it directly with the microscope.

561 Torsion of the testis (3621) with infarction in a 13-year-old boy who complained of pain and swelling for two weeks which settled and then recurred two days before operation, when the spermatic cord was found to be twisted and the testis (3.5×2.5×2cm) and epididymis plum-coloured and infarcted. This was confirmed histologically. Maldescent, unduly broad mesorchium (bell-clapper testis) or presence of tumour may predispose to torsion. The mechanism is not always clear but the condition may be bilateral so that prophylactic orchidopexy is often worthwhile.

562

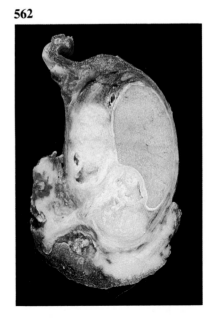

562 Tuberculous epididymitis (4455) in a 42-year-old man with a discharging sinus on the right scrotum. The specimen is a swollen testis (7×5×4cm) with a 5cm length of cord and attached piece of scrotal skin bearing a sinus communicating with pus-filled cavities in the epididymis. The testis is uninvolved. Sections showed appearances of caseating tuberculosis with demonstrable AAFB.

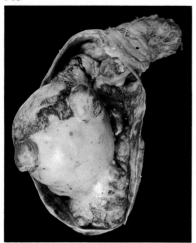

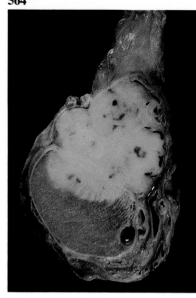

563 Yolk-sac tumour of the testis (orchioblastoma) (8003) from a 31-year-old man on treatment for Behçet's disease for years – drugs included prednisolone and cyclophosphamide. He developed an acute hydrocoele and an enlarged testis ($10 \times 7 \times 6\,cm$) was removed. It was largely replaced by white and yellow neoplasm partly solid, partly cystic and with many areas of haemorrhage and necrosis. Nodules of neoplasm are present on the tunica vaginalis posteriorly and at the upper pole. Sections showed appearances of malignant testicular neoplasm resembling that seen in yolk-sac tumour of children, with proliferating cells ranging from squames to cuboidal, columnar to polyhedral, in solid trabecular and alveolar and acinar arrangements often with perivascular mantles. There was abundant alpha-feto-protein demonstrable by immunoperoxidase technique.

564 Malignant lymphoma of the left testis (8006) in a 75-year-old man treated two years earlier for reticulum-cell sarcoma (malignant histiocytic lymphoma) of the tonsil with radiotherapy; then had enlarged inguinal nodes showing similar histopathological appearances; now complaining of swollen testis. It is ($6 \times 4 \times 4\,cm$) with a hard pale mass ($4 \times 3 \times 3\,cm$) at its upper pole. Sections showed appearances of malignant histiocytic lymphoma. Seminoma is very rare at this age. Electron-micrographically the cells showed no obvious epithelial characteristics.

565 Leukaemic infiltration of the testis (8006) in a child on treatment for acute lymphoblastic leukaemia. The section shows immature testicular tubules separated by dense round-cell infiltrate, including large lymphoblastic cells and small lymphocytes. Both testes were affected. *(H&E × 83)*

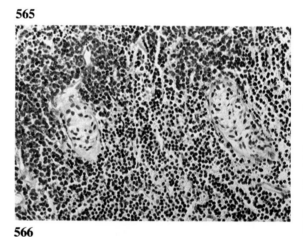

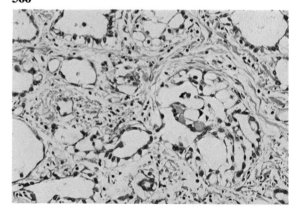

566 Adenomatoid tumour of the testis (9050) A 2cm nodule removed from the testis of a 30-year-old man. Section shows characteristic spaces lined by vacuolated cells. The lesion is of uncertain origin but benign. *(H&E × 83)*

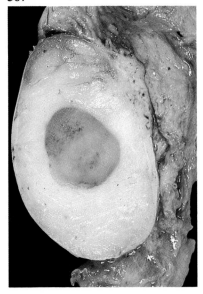

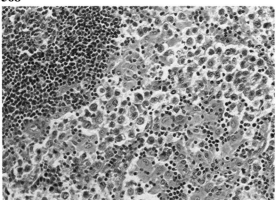

568 Seminoma of the testis (9063) Section of lesion shown in **567** shows clumps of large polygonal cells with pale staining cytoplasm and brisk epithelioid cell and lymphocytic infiltrate in the stroma. *(H&E × 53)*

567 Seminoma of the testis (9063) removed one week after laparotomy for retroperitoneal tumour thought to be sarcoma. The pathologist diagnosed metastatic seminoma: the left testis was found to feel slightly firmer than the right, and was excised. The specimen consisted of 14 cm of cord and testis (4 × 2.5 × 2 cm) with much of it replaced by seminoma, leaving a small central brownish area and a narrow rim of unaffected testicular tissue at the upper pole. The patient, aged 29 years, responded excellently to radiotherapy and chemotherapy.

569

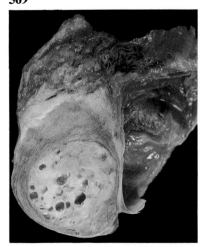

569 Teratoma of the testis (9081) from a 65-year-old man who complained of swelling of the scrotum for 10 months. The mass was painful on palpation and partly transilluminatable. At operation there was a large hydrocoele and a testis of near normal size (4.5 × 3.5 × 2.5 cm), but on transverse slicing a hard greyish-blue, partly cystic spherical mass was revealed within the testis. Histologically the appearances were those of a differentiated teratoma with bone, brain, mature cartilage, collagen, cysts lined by tall columnar, cuboidal or flattened squamous cells and containing keratin or mucin. The seminiferous tubules showed partial atrophy in keeping with the patient's age.

570

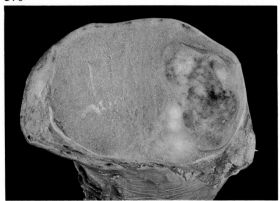

571

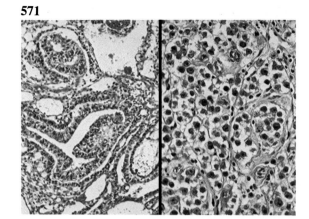

570 Combined seminoma (9063) **and teratoma** (9083) **(embryonal carcinoma)** (9083) from a 33-year-old man who complained of swelling of the testis for 10 months. The enlarged testis (6×3.5×3cm) has in its lower half (on right) a soft neoplastic mass (3×2cm) comprising a larger darker haemorrhagic portion and a smaller paler whitish cream-coloured mass (10×5mm). The rest of the testis and epididymis appear normal. Sections showed seminoma and highly cellular undifferentiated teratoma (embryonal carcinoma) without trophoblast.

571 Combined seminoma (9063) **and teratoma of the testis** (9083) Section of lesion shown in **570** to show on right seminoma and on left embryonal carcinoma. *(H&E×53, ×83)*

572

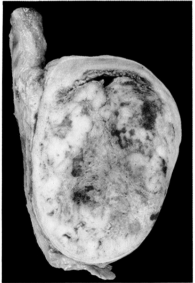

572 Undifferentiated teratoma of testis (embryonal carcinoma) (9083) The enlarged (9×6×6cm) testis weighs 200g: it is more or less replaced by grey, partly necrotic and haemorrhagic neoplasm showing appearances of embryonal carcinoma.

573

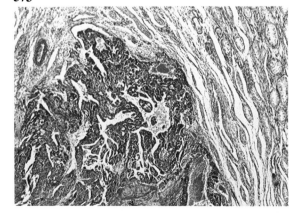

573 Chorioncarcinoma of the testis (9083) Section showing both cytotrophoblast (Langhans' cells) and syncytiotrophoblast infiltrating testicular tissues. The patient presented with haemoptysis caused by metastases in the lungs. The urine contained large amounts of chorionic gonadotropin. *(H&E×33)*

8   Female genitalia

Vulva (T80)

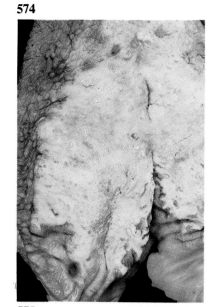

574

574   Leukoplakia of the vulva (7361) from a 78-year-old woman with an intractable itch. A biopsy three months earlier was reported as showing epithelial hyperplasia with acanthosis, hyperkeratosis, parakeratosis and much chronic inflammatory cell infiltrate in the connective tissues, appearances in keeping with the clinical diagnosis of leukoplakia. No evidence of malignancy was seen. The same changes were evident in the vulvectomy specimen (7×6cm) with much of the surface prominently indurated and white.

575

575   Leukoplakia of the vulva (7361) from a 46-year-old nulliparous woman who complained of itch and swelling of the left labium majus. A (2×1.5cm) piece of labium has white plaques on it and sections were reported as showing hyperkeratosis, areas of intra-epithelial carcinoma showing an extraordinary mitotic activity (75 per HP field) and some irregular pleomorphic squamous-cell downgrowths which warrant a diagnosis of superficial infiltrating squamous-cell carcinoma. Section shows hyperkeratosis, nuclear pleomorphism and dense subepithelial round-cell infiltrate. *(H&E×53)*

576

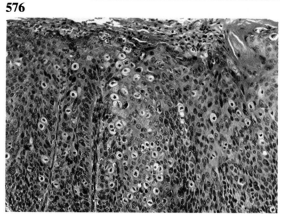

576   Leukoplakia of the vulva (7361) Same specimen as in **575**. Section shows parakeratosis and disorderly arrangement of epithelial cells and 70 mitoses in this field. *(H&E×83)*

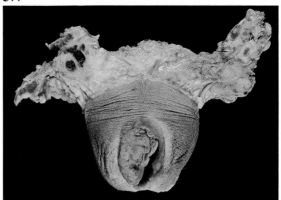

577 Squamous-cell carcinoma of the vulva (8073) from a 70-year-old woman with a large (5×3.5cm) ulcerated tumour on the right side extending into the vagina. Inguinal nodes on both sides were enlarged by metastases.

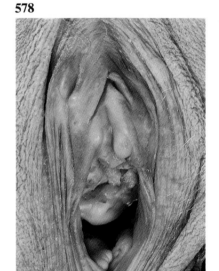

578 Squamous-cell carcinoma of the clitoris (8073) from a 79-year-old woman who complained of something coming down the vagina. A mass (5×4×3cm) involving clitoris, vagina and urethra showed appearance of well-differentiated squamous-cell carcinoma.

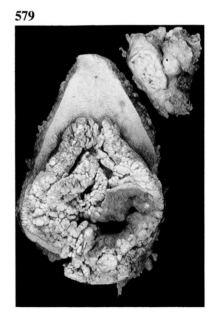

579 Squamous-cell carcinoma of the vulva (8073) complicating extensive condylomata from a 42-year-old woman who had suffered from 'warts' for 10 years. The left vulva had become ulcerated and lumps appeared in the groins. A radical vulvectomy with node dissection of left inguinal region was carried out. The specimen shows labia and adjacent skin covered with innumerable warty masses ranging in size from a few millimetres to several centimetres tall, generally smooth and pointed (giant condyloma acuminatum). A (7.5×4cm) malignant ulcer with deep (3cm) crater is present on the left side and involves the clitoris. Sections confirmed the diagnosis of squamous-cell carcinoma arising in giant condylomata acuminata. The nodes in the groin were more or less replaced by metastases. Perianal warts also removed at this time showed changes of in-situ carcinoma.

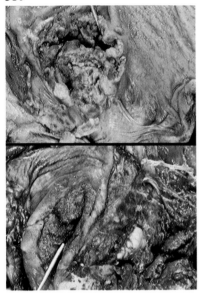

Vagina (T81)

580 Rectovaginal fistula (4631) in a
71-year-old woman with a carcinoma
of the anus. The probe passes from the
ulcerated carcinoma (of basaloid type)
of the anus through vaginal wall to
emerge in the floor of an ovoid ulcer
(3 × 1 cm).

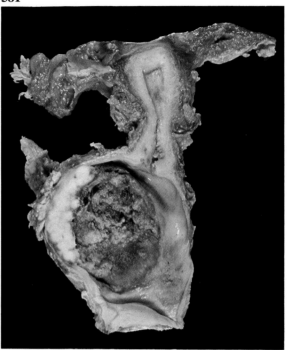

581 Squamous-cell carcinoma of the vagina (8073)
from a 72-year-old woman who complained of vaginal
discharge. Biopsy of a circular (8 × 6 cm) ulcer on
posterior vaginal wall was reported as squamous-cell
carcinoma with numerous eosinophil polymorphonuclear leucocytes in the stroma. A posterior exenteration for primary vaginal carcinoma was carried out.
Metastases were present in lymph nodes removed from
parametrium and right external iliac regions. No
evidence was present of uterine or anorectal carcinoma.

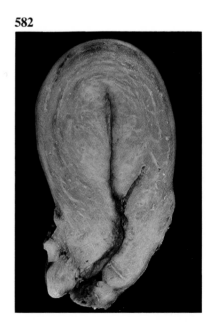

Uterus (T82)

582 False passage (1000) created at curettage before
hysterectomy and posterior colporrhaphy, in a 43-year-
old multiparous 5:2 woman. The uterus is big (10 × 7 ×
5.5) with body bent backwards (retroverted) on the
cervix. A longitudinal slice showed blood in the
endometrial cavity and in a false passage leading
upwards and anteriorly for 2 cm. The only histological
feature of note was adenomyosis.

583

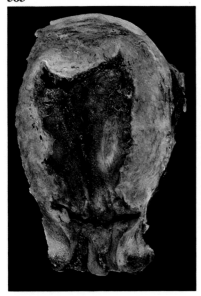

584

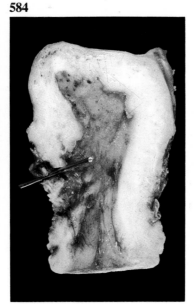

585

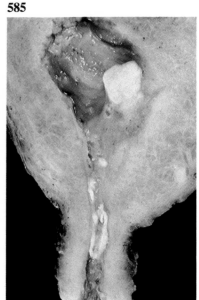

583 Lacerated cervix (1000) at attempted forceps delivery of a 23-year-old woman eventually delivered by caesarean section, then sterilised by subtotal hysterectomy. The bulky (17 × 12 × 9 cm) supracervical uterus has a triangular laceration 5 cm long, 2.5 cm at its widest tapering to 1 cm where it meets the lower segment scar. The uterine cavity shows the expected haemorrhagic placental bed.

584 Perforated uterus (1000) 15 days after suction termination in a 27-year-old woman with history of bleeding on two occasions after the abortion; 3.3 cm above the cervix a 10 mm wide passage extends postero-laterally and shows much haemorrhage into the uterine wall. Histologically there was chronic inflammatory change in the area of perforation and in the retained placental tissues in the right cornu.

585 Post-irradiation scar in the endocervix of the uterus (1130) showing residual carcinosarcoma from a woman of 58 years. She had been treated with intracavity radium two months earlier after complaining of post-menopausal bleeding; the cytology smear had been reported as showing malignant cells. The uterus was bulky (12 × 10 × 8 cm) and filled with golden-yellow fluid. A white nodule 2 × 2 × 1.5 cm of residual neoplasm (histologically viable) is seen projecting from the wall which shows thickening with whorled appearance caused by adenomyosis. The right ovary contained a fibroma and the left a papillary cystadenocarcinoma.

586

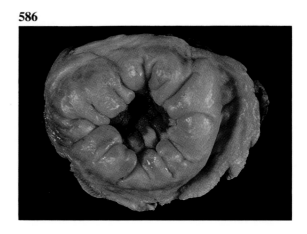

586 Post-cone cervical scarring (1512) in a 40-year-old woman who had a cone biopsy done two months previously for early invasive carcinoma. At hysterectomy the cervix showed radiating grooves but no residual carcinoma.

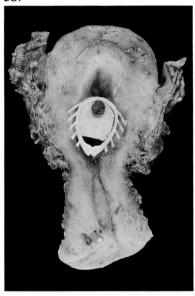

587 Intrauterine contraceptive device (3200) in a bulky uterus (10×5×5cm) from a 42-year-old woman who complained of menorrhagia for 12 years.

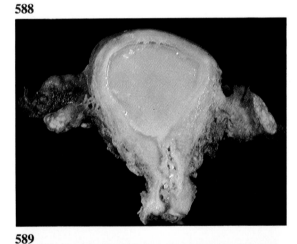

588 Pyometra (4046) in a 56-year-old woman with carcinoma of the uterine cervix treated with radium 10 weeks before extended hysterectomy. The dilated (5cm) uterine cavity is filled with foul-smelling, greenish-yellow pus. The site of irradiation in the endocervical canal is pale yellowish-white but necrosis extends down into the vaginal cuff. No residual carcinoma was identified. There was severe chronic salpingo-oöphoritis with serosal adhesions.

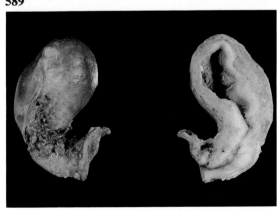

589 Tuberculosis of the uterus (4470) from a 77-year-old woman. The whole of the endometrial cavity is lined by tuberculous granulation tissue and many AAFB were demonstrable in the granulomatous lesions. Both fallopian tubes and ovaries were involved.

590

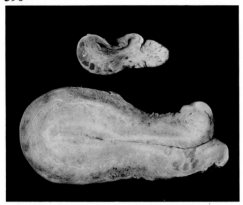

591

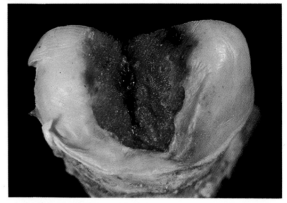

592

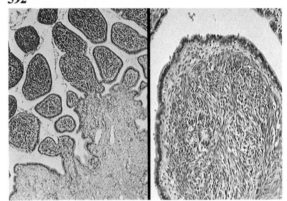

593

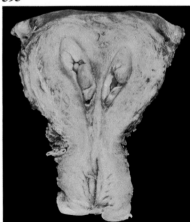

594

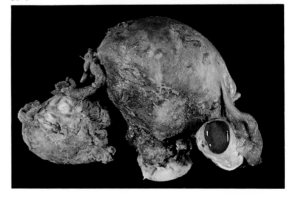

590 Cervical erosion (4610) from a woman who complained of menor- rhagia and vaginal discharge. Hysterectomy was done: the uterus (10×6×4.5cm) has a bulky (3×3cm) cervix with lips showing 'erosion' for about 1cm round the os. There was a small adenofibroma of the left ovary.

591 Cervical erosion (4610) Close-up of the cervix from same specimen as in **590** to show red granular lips.

592 Cervical erosion (4610) Same specimen as in **590**. Section to show, on left, superficial polypoid granu- lations packed with plasma cells and covered with columnar cuboidal epithelium; on the right, adeno- fibroma of the ovary with fibrous stroma covered with epithelium, which in places resembles that of fallopian tube. *(H&E×33, ×53)*

593 Bicornuate uterus with endometrial hyperplasia (7300) from a 29-year-old woman who complained of menorrhagia. The bulky uterus (11×8.5×4cm) with attached cervix (3.5×3cm) has a 1cm slit and polypoid endometrium lining the two cavities. Histologically the appearances were those of cystic hyperplasia with polyposis, some adenomyosis and there was cervical endometriosis.

594 Endometriosis (7671) **and adenomyoma of the uterus** (7672) from a 49-year-old woman who com- plained of menorrhagia and intermittent pain in both iliac fossae. Para 4/0. At hysterectomy there were adhesions over most of the pelvic organs and the uterine enlargement (13×10×9cm) was caused largely by a fundal adenomyoma. The right ovary contains a 2.5cm in diameter 'chocolate cyst' (endometrial cyst).

595   Metastatic carcinoma in the uterus (8016) from a 63-year-old woman with a long history of postmenopausal bleeding. The specimen includes uterus (9×4×4cm) with both tubes and ovaries, the left being enlarged (5×5cm) by neoplasm: mucoid carcinoma replaces much of the lower uterine wall and upper endocervix and projects posteriorly having penetrated the myometrium. In this case the problem is deciding which lesion is the primary – the presence of calcispheres in the lesions favoured ovary. The endometrium was atrophic and the cervix chronically inflamed.

595

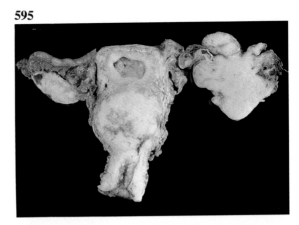

596

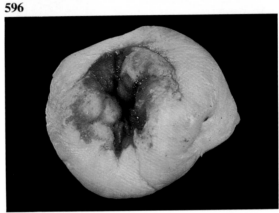

596   Carcinoma in situ of the cervix uteri (8072) from a 29-year-old woman who requested sterilisation by hysterectomy after a cervical smear was reported positive Class V and biopsy reported as carcinoma in situ. The cervix of the uterus is 3.5×2cm and its lips show fine nodularity and red granular areas of erosion. It was blocked in 14 pieces and sections showed squamocolumnar junction in 12. Histologically there was a ring of dysplasia merging into undifferentiated carcinoma in situ, with glandular extension excision being complete.

597

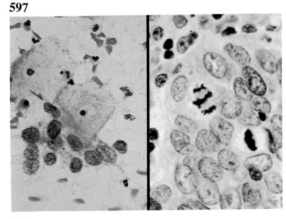

597   Carcinoma in situ (8072) Class V smear from same patient as in **596** and on right section of biopsy showing three group metaphase alongside prophase mitotic figure in undifferentiated in situ carcinomatous epithelium. *(Papanicolau ×133) (H&E ×330)*

598

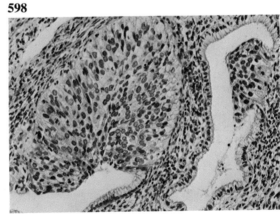

598   Carcinoma in situ (8072) with glandular extension: same case as in **596**. *(H&E ×83)*

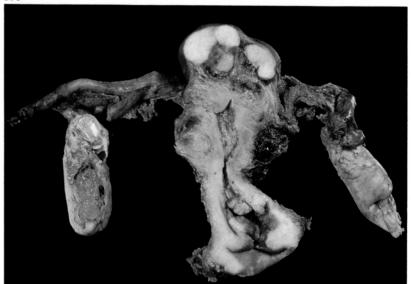

599 Endocervical squamous-cell carcinoma (8073) from a 67-year-old woman with post-menopausal bleeding and Class IV smear. Biopsy showed squamous-cell carcinoma. Hysterectomy specimen shows the neoplasm 3cm long beginning at external os and extending upwards involving all of a 1cm zone anteriorly. The uterus was enlarged ($11 \times 6 \times 5$cm) by fibroids and the ovaries contained chocolate cysts.

600

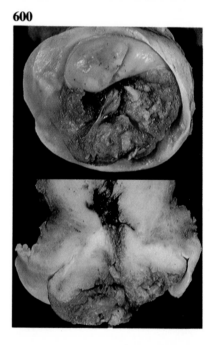

600 Fungating squamous-cell carcinoma (8073) of the cervix of a 43-year-old woman who had a cone biopsy (18 months before) after two Class IV smears. The ($10 \times 5 \times 3$cm) uterus was excised with a 1.5cm vaginal cuff. On the left the 4.2cm diameter cervix shows 60 per cent replacement by friable squamous carcinoma, histologically of well-differentiated keratinising squamous-cell type. Ulceration in the vaginal cuff is caused by metastases. On the right the cervix has been sliced transversely to show a wedge of malignant tissue corresponding to the cone biopsy carried out 18 months earlier. The endocervical glands are cystic.

601

601 Adenocarcinoma of the endometrium (8143) from a 77-year-old woman with post-menopausal bleeding. Curettage produced a large quantity of friable tissue reported as well-differentiated glandular carcinoma of the endometrium. The uterus ($10 \times 6 \times 5$cm) has a dilated cavity (diameter 4.5cm) filled with papillary neoplasm which replaces nearly all of the endometrium and invades myometrium to within a millimetre on the lateral aspect. Histologically the papillary adenocarcinoma was highly cellular (up to 15 mitoses per HP field including abnormal forms). The remaining endometrium was atrophic but showed cystic glands. The ovaries and lymph nodes removed from pelvic wall were free of neoplasm.

602 Adenocarcinoma of the endometrium (8143)
Section from the case shown in **601**. On the left a solid
area showing closely packed columnar cells forming
acini: nuclei are hyperchromatic and several mitotic
figures are included in the field. On the right a papillary
area showing aggregates of large histiocytes with pale
staining granular cytoplasm. *(H&E × 53, × 83)*

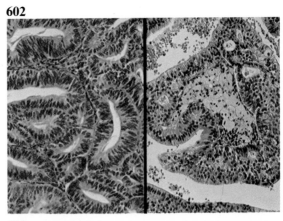

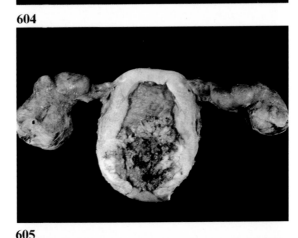

603 Adenocarcinoma of the uterus (8143) from a 76-
year-old woman with post-menopausal bleeding and
Class V smear. The bulky uterus (9 × 6 × 6 cm) has an
enlarged cavity filled by papillary and solid whitish-
yellow neoplasm originating from endometrium over a
wide area except for short lengths on the left lower and
upper right wall. It is only superficially invasive but
invasion of vessels was seen in a block from posterior
fundus. The sections of the ovaries (each 3 × 2 × 1.5 cm)
showed them to be free of metastases but their stroma
was unusually cellular.

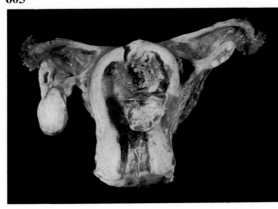

604 Adenocarcinoma of the uterus (8143) from 66-
year-old woman Para 2/0 who complained of post-
menopausal bleeding. Curettage produced friable
carcinomatous fragments. The uterus is greatly swollen
10 × 6 × 5 cm. Papillary adenocarcinoma involves the
lower half of the cavity, penetrates myometrium and
infiltrates the upper endocervix. Cellular foci on the
surface of the ovaries were regarded as serosal hyperplastic inclusions rather than metastases. There is
bilateral pyosalpinx.

605 Endometrial cystadenomatous polyp (8210),
endometrial hyperplasia (7300) and **endometrial carcinoma** (8143) **associated with ovarian thecoma** (8600)
in a 73-year-old woman. A (9 × 6 × 5 cm) uterus, an
enlarged (4 × 2 × 1.7 cm) left ovary and two separate
neoplastic masses in the dilated uterine cavity. An
upper irregular necrotic and brown carcinoma which
penetrates the myometrium near the right cornu, and
lower down a cystic mass with smooth surface dipping
into the internal os. Histologically the carcinoma was
of columnar-cell type with anaplastic polyhedral cell
foci and clear-cell areas. Some endometrial glands were
lined by epithelium similar to that of the neoplasm
producing appearances of an in situ carcinoma.

606

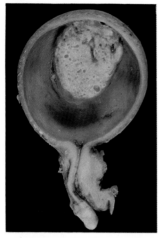

607

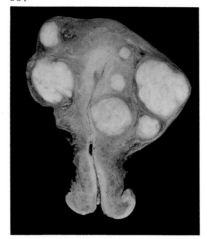

608

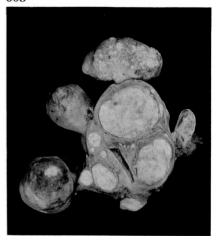

606 Endometrial adenomatous polyp (8210) from a 76-year-old woman with post-menopausal bleeding. Curettage a week before hysterectomy produced curettings which were reported as showing adenocarcinoma. The hysterectomy specimen was a bulky uterus ($10 \times 7 \times 7$ cm) with cavity filled with blood clot and at the fundus a polypoid (4×4 cm) mass with cystic cut surface. Histologically it is a benign cystic endometrial polyp. There was no residual carcinoma in sections from many blocks of endometrium which appeared generally atrophic. However, the ovaries and nodules on the serosa both showed infiltration by adeno-carcinoma like that seen in the endometrial curettage. It was felt that the curettage had pro-bably removed all of the endo-metrial primary.

607 'Fibroids' (fibroleiomyomata) of the uterus (8890) from a 47-year-old woman with longstanding menor-rhagia since the delivery of her first child by caesarean section. The uterus is enlarged ($12 \times 10 \times 7$ cm) as a result of multiple fibroids up to 4 cm in diameter: they are situated in sub-serous, submucous and interstitial locations. All were histologically benign.

608 'Fibroids' (fibroleiomyomata) of the uterus (8890) from a 48-year-old doctor, a spinster, who complained of irregular bleeding and was found to have a large irregular pelvic mass. Hysterectomy specimen weighs 1,600 g. The fibroids varied greatly in size, the largest being 10 cm in diameter. A pedunculated one at the fundus was heavily calcified.

609

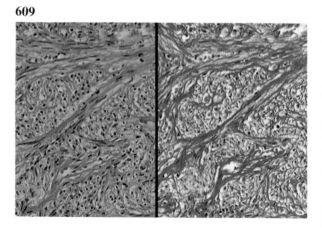

609 Fibroid of the uterus (8890) Section of one of the lesions shown in **608**. The cut surface showed a watered silk appearance caused by the interlacing of bundles of muscle and fibrous tissue. On the left stained H&E on the right van Gieson with which collagen stains red and muscle yellow-brown. *(×53)*

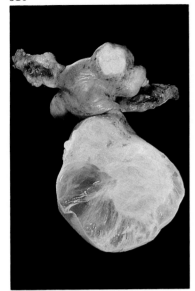

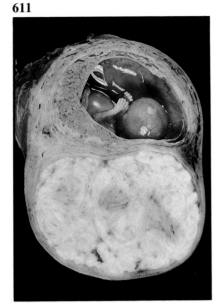

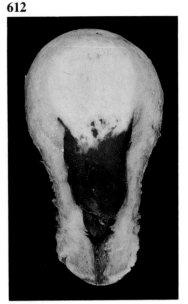

610 **Cystic and myxomatous degeneration** (8890) in a fibroid from a 75-year-old spinster with a ten-year history of an abdominal swelling. The largest subserous fibroid (10cm diameter) showed degeneration (cystic and mucoid) on histological section but no evidence of malignancy.

611 **Red degeneration in a fibroid** (8890) in a pregnant uterus. The 36-year-old woman presented with abdominal swelling, nausea and vomiting having missed two periods. The uterus (17 × 12 × 12cm) is distorted by fibroids and by swelling caused by a normal gestation sac containing a 6cm long (CR) normal foetus. The serosal surface was studded with tiny tubercles caused by deciduosis. The largest fibroid shows 'red degeneration'.

612 **Stromal sarcoma of the endometrium** (8933) in a nulliparous 41-year-old woman who complained of menorrhagia. The uterus is big (12 × 6 × 5cm), of regular shape but the cavity is filled with a pale neoplasm (4 × 3.5cm) and blood clot. There is infiltration of myometrium to within 3mm of serosa by the neoplasm which histologically was reported as stromal sarcoma. Three years later there was recurrence of sarcoma on the peritoneum with malignant ascites.

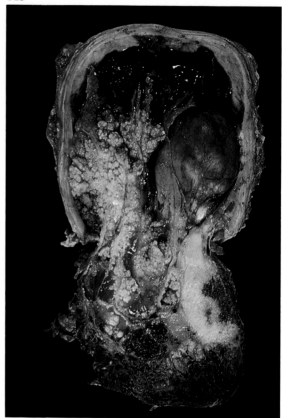

613

613 Carcinosarcoma of the endometrium (8983) from a 65-year-old woman who complained of two weeks abdominal pain and swelling of the abdomen. The uterus felt like an 18-weeks gestation. Necrotic tissue was found in the vagina and a dark-red mass with white papillary projections lay in the dilated cervical canal. Bloody fluid and clots issued from the uterine cavity in which a (18 × 11 × 10cm) neoplasm could be seen arising from the lower half of the right and almost the whole of the breadth of the posterior walls. There were ovoid yellow masses in the upper part, grey solid areas in the lower half and numerous papillary masses and blood clot free in the cavity. Sections showed varied histological appearances but essentially those of carcinosarcoma (malignant mixed mesodermal tumour) with predominance of sarcomatous elements.

614

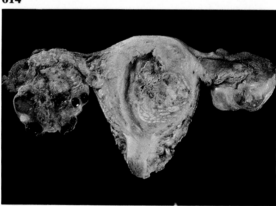

614 Chorioncarcinoma of the uterus (9103) from a 25-year-old woman admitted as threatened abortion but uterus small for dates and Hb 40 per cent. Chest xray showed opacities in the left lung field. Curettage produced cheesy necrotic material which histologically was reported as chorionepithelioma. Hysterectomy (in 1956) was done: the uterus is moderately enlarged, the roughly spherical body having a diameter of 8cm. The posterior wall is expanded by neoplasm which replaces the whole thickness of myometrium and has a mottled white cut surface. Both ovaries are enlarged and of polycystic contour; a large mass on the right mesovarium is a metastasis.

615

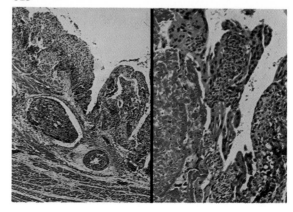

615 Chorioncarcinoma of the uterus (9103) Section of the lesion shown in **614**. On the left the endometrium is replaced by carcinoma showing syncytiotrophoblast and cytotrophoblast. A large vascular sinus contains neoplasm. On the right section to show syncytiotrophoblast, cytotrophoblast and necrosis. *(H&E × 33, × 53)*

Fallopian tube (T86)

616   Ectopic pregnancy (2620) in rudimentary horn of the uterus of a 24-year-old woman Para 1/0 with three months amenorrhoea and vaginal bleeding for three days. The specimen consists of apparently normal right tube and ovary alongside which there is a spheroid mass 4cm in diameter) nine-tenths covered with serosa. The isthmic end of the tube appears to enter the mass but no lumen could be identified. On slicing, a gestation sac containing a tiny 2mm embryo is revealed, surrounded by muscle (4 to 8mm thick).

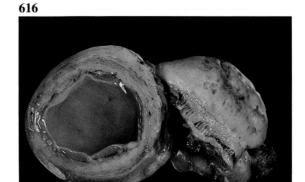

617   Ectopic pregnancy (2620) in fallopian tube from a 32-year-old woman para 2/0. The fimbrial end of the tube is distended by a mass (4 × 2.5 × 2cm) which on section shows appearances of ruptured ectopic tubal pregnancy as evidenced by chorionic villi and trophoblast. The ovary contains a corpus luteum of pregnancy. The endometrium was in secretory phase – and certainly not overtly to be recognised as coming from a pregnant patient.

617
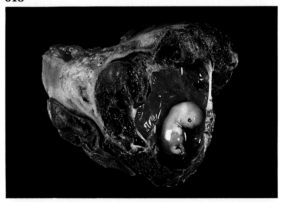

618   Ectopic pregnancy (2620) Tubal abortion from a 29-year-old woman para 1/1 complaining of central abdominal pain and ten weeks amenorrhoea followed by vaginal bleeding. The (8 × 6 × 4cm) mass includes an intact gestation sac (4.5cm in diameter) containing a 2.3cm apparently normal embryo.

618
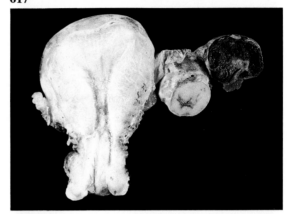

619   Ruptured tubal pregnancy (2620) with normal foetus. The woman was admitted as an emergency with signs of gross intraperitoneal haemorrhage: she was sixteen weeks pregnant and at laparotomy the 22mm long foetus was found alongside the ruptured isthmus of fallopian tube.

619
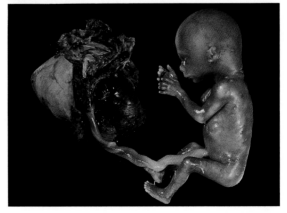

620 Hydrosalpinx (2620) from a 23-year-old woman requesting sterilisation. The right 6 cm long fallopian tube was chronically inflamed with appearances of salpingitis isthmica nodosa. The left (15 cm long) fallopian tube is thin walled and retort shaped, filled with watery fluid. Sections showed continuing inflammation in the wall.

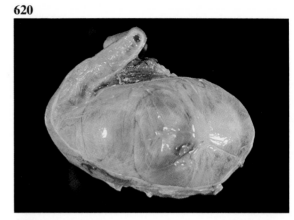

621 Pyosalpinx (4046) from a 33-year-old woman complaining of abdominal pain for 2 days – she gave a history of previous pelvic inflammation and at laparotomy both fallopian tubes and ovaries were inflamed. The left tube was 10 cm long, dilated (1.5 cm) and filled with pus. The right tube is 10 cm long dilated and filled with pus firmly attached to the 3 cm long ovary forming a tubo-ovarian abscess.

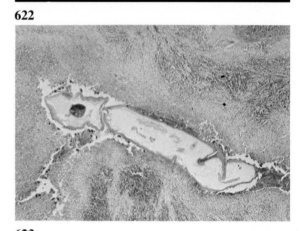

622 Threadworm tubo-ovarian granuloma (4400) presenting as an acute abdominal emergency in a 19-year-old spinster, one of a family of four. She had had her vermiform appendix removed two years earlier. Ectopic pregnancy was thought possible and at laparotomy the whole pelvis was a mass of adhesions and tuberculosis was thought likely. A left tubo-ovarian mass ($8 \times 4 \times 3$ cm) was removed and the most striking feature histologically was widespread granulomatous inflammation with dense eosinophil polymorphonuclear leucocytic infiltration and Charcot-Leyden crystal formation. Altogether five gravid female threadworms were identified in tracks in tube wall and ovary. Section shows one of these cut slightly askew: the oesophageal bulb is seen at the head end (left) and lateral cuticular crests are visible where the worm is bent on itself. There is much necrosis of adjacent granulation tissue which is packed with chronic inflammatory cells. Diagnostic eggs lie free among the exudate; some are phagocytosed and others appear covered with a calcific coat (see **623**). A clear-adhesive-tape swab of perianal tissue was positive for threadworm eggs and her blood film showed eosinophilia. She has remained infertile since. *(H&E × 13)*

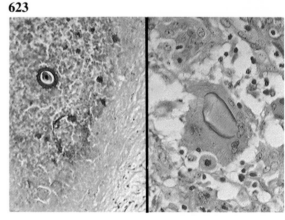

623 Threadworm tubo-ovarian granuloma (4400) Same case as **622**. Section shows on right multinucleate macrophage with ingested threadworm egg shell stained with phloxine: on the left granulomatous lesion with calcified coating of threadworm egg. *(H&E × 53, H. Phloxine-T × 133)*

624 **Papillary adenocarcinoma of fallopian tube** (8143) from a 61-year-old woman complaining of post menopausal bleeding. Hysterectomy and bilateral salpingo-oöphorectomy was carried out. The right tube was normal, the left is dilated in its distal half to 2 cm diameter and its lumen is filled with papillary neoplasm which appears to arise from the mucosa of the ampulla. Histologically it was a well-differentiated papillary adenocarcinoma showing much mitotic activity and nuclear pleomorphism. Both ovaries and endometrium were atrophic.

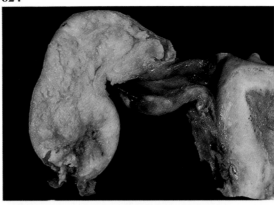

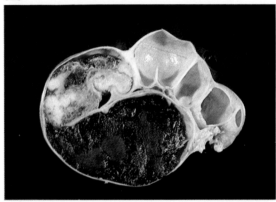

625 **Sarcoma of fallopian tube** (8803) This dilated (9 × 6 cm) fallopian tube appeared dark red at laparotomy and was thought to be an ectopic pregnancy or haematosalpinx. On section the (5 × 3 cm) fleshy neoplasm which fills the lumen proximal to the haematoma showed appearances of a spindle-cell sarcoma.

Ovary (T87)

626 **Ectopic pregnancy in ovary** (2620) from a 32-year-old woman. The enlarged ovary (5 × 5 × 3 cm) has an almost spherical (4 cm) mass consisting of coagulated blood, laminated and surrounding a sac with crenulated walls and pale flecks of tissue at its periphery, and a corpus luteum at one pole. Only a few well preserved chorionic villi remained in the ectopic pregnancy.

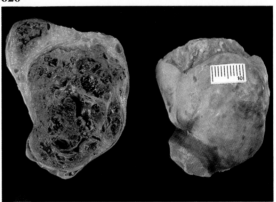

627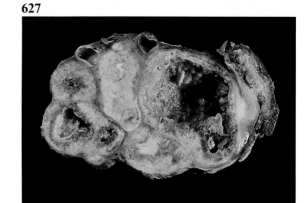

627   Tubo-ovarian abscess (4174) from a 29-year-old woman with recurrent abdominal pain and with (10 × 6 × 5 cm) tubo-ovarian mass which on section shows abscess cavities filled with green pus.

628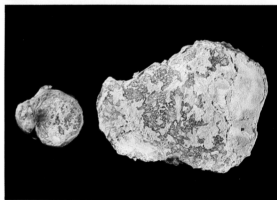

628   Ossified fibromas of right ovary (7655) from an 83-year-old woman with abdominal distension due to a huge (22 cm diameter) but benign left ovarian cyst of mixed mucinous and serous papilligerous type weighing 1,900 g. The right ovary felt like a stone and required a diamond saw to make a cross section in which the calcified and osseous tissue appear white and brown respectively.

629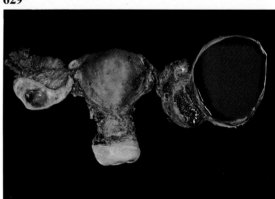

629   Endometrial cysts of ovaries (7671) from a 40-year-old woman – Para 2/0. They were removed at hysterectomy and bilateral salpingo-oöphorectomy when, two months after appendicectomy, she complained of continuing pain in the RIF. The uterus is enlarged (10 × 6 × 6 cm) and there are chocolate (endometrial) cysts in both ovaries, that on the right being 8 cm diameter.

630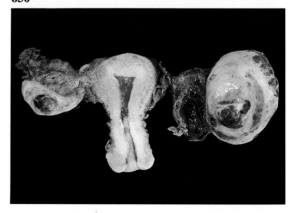

630   Endometrial cysts of ovaries (7671) Same specimen as **629** to show walls of the endometrial cysts after removal of contents and opened uterus.

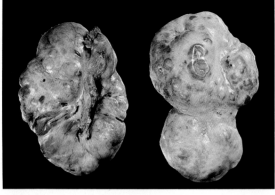

631

631 Krukenberg tumours of the ovaries (8016) from a 36-year-old woman with an annular adenocarcinoma of sigmoid colon found to have malignant ascites and enlarged ovaries retaining their ovarian shape, mainly solid and histologically infiltrated by highly cellular polyhedral cell carcinoma. Krukenberg tumours are usually associated with gastric mucin secreting carcinoma.

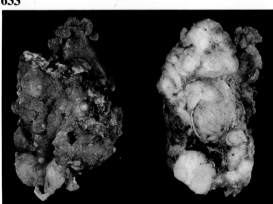

632

632 Krukenberg tumours of ovaries (8016) Same case as **631** to show cut surface. There are one or two small cysts so that one could argue that these were second primary carcinomas of ovary rather than metastases but on balance the latter diagnosis was preferred.

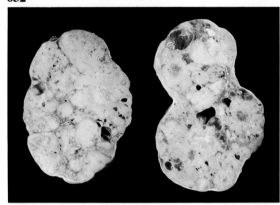

633

633 Bilateral primary ovarian carcinoma (8443) of ovary: each is replaced by mainly solid adenocarcinoma forming irregular masses ($7 \times 5 \times 4$cm).

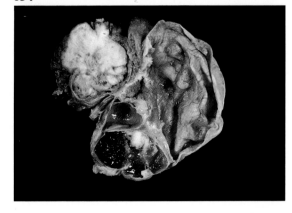

634

634 Cystic and solid carcinomas of ovary from a 52-year-old woman complaining of dyspareunia and pain in RIF. The right ovary is large ($12 \times 8 \times 8$cm) with cystic part thin walled and multiloculate with papilligerous lining with thick areas up to 2cm, while the solid (6cm diameter) part is soft and nodular. Histologically the appearances were reported as papillary serous cystadenocarcinoma of ovary. There was direct spread to the omentum.

635

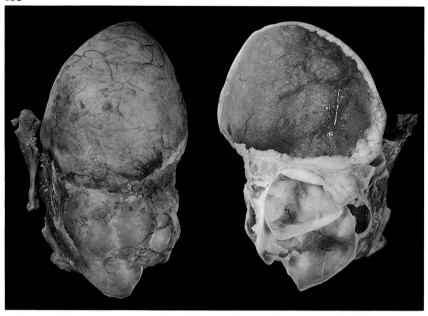

635 Serous cystadenoma (papilligerous) of ovary
(8143) from a 34-year-old woman complaining of
abdominal swelling. A hysterectomy and bilateral
salpingo-oöphorectomy was done: both ovaries were
replaced by cysts – right ($20 \times 16 \times 14$ cm) and left
($10 \times 8 \times 7$ cm) containing serous fluid and showing

inner wall studded with papillary masses ranging in size
from 1 mm to 5 cm. There were papilligerous projections on the serosal surface. Histologically the lesions
were reported as cellular papilligerous serous cyst-
adenomas.

636

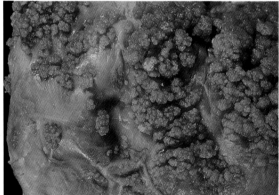

**636 Papilligerous serous cystadenocarcinoma of the
ovary** (8460) from a 71-year-old woman Para 5/0. She
complained of abdominal swelling and discomfort. The
right ovary is replaced by a large 16cm diameter
triloculate cystic mass showing papilligerous projections
lining the largest loculus, forming quite thick solid
masses and also spreading over part of the adjacent
serosal surface. The other ovary and endometrium
appeared atrophic.

637

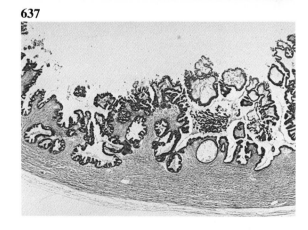

**637 Papilligerous serous cystadenocarcinoma of the
ovary** (8463) Section of a lesion shown in **636**. The
papillary processes are lined by multilayered cuboidal
cells with hyperchromatic pleomorphic nuclei, showing
mitotic activity, and in places there are calcispheres in
the stroma. *(H&E × 13)*

638

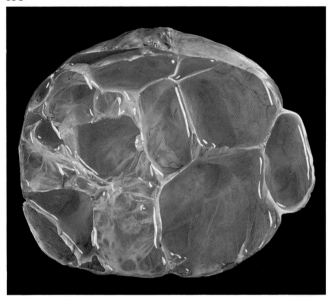

638 Mucinous cystadenoma of the ovary (8470) from a 63-year-old woman Para 2/0 with abdominal swelling. The right ovary is replaced by a 16cm in diameter multiloculated cystic mass with smooth serosal surface and mucin-containing loculi up to 10cm in diameter. The walls are thin, nowhere showing any suspicion of malignancy. The uterus was 9 × 5 × 4cm with endometrium showing cystic hyperplasia. The left ovary was atrophic. Virtually any lesion of the ovary appears capable of stimulating endometrial hyperplasia, in this case the presence of the mucinous cyst is an acceptable cause. The contents of the cyst are precipitable with alcohol but not with acetic acid, hence the usage of the term pseudomucinous cystadenoma by some pathologists.

639

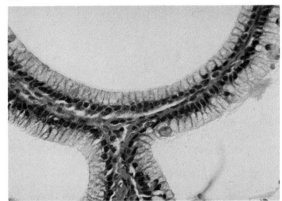

639 Mucinous cystadenoma of the ovary (8470) Section of a lesion shown in **638** to show tall columnar mucin-secreting cells with nuclei situated near the base of the cells. *(H&E × 133)*

640 Cystadenoma (multiloculate) of the right ovary (8463) from a 71-year-old woman on chemotherapy for breast cancer. It is 17 × 15 × 10cm and weighs 1350g. Histologically it is a benign mucin-secreting cystadenoma.

640

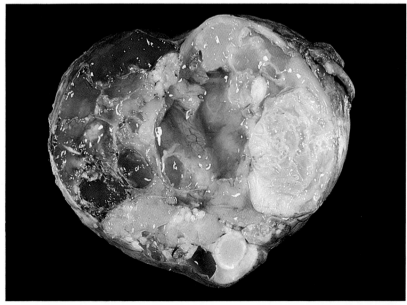

641 **Thecoma of the ovary** (8470) from an 87-year-old woman with cystic endometrial hyperplasia. She had complained for years of abdominal discomfort. The tumour weighed 965 g, was 20 cm across, with one half showing solid yellow and white cut surface, while the other half was cystic with myxomatous stroma. Frozen (cryostat) section demonstrated abundant lipid (sudanophilic and birefringent) in the cytoplasm of the cells, establishing the diagnosis of thecoma. The other ovary contained a small 3 cm in diameter adenofibroma.

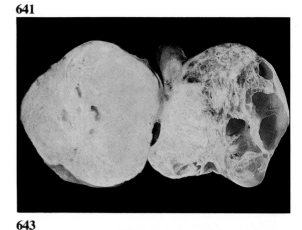
641

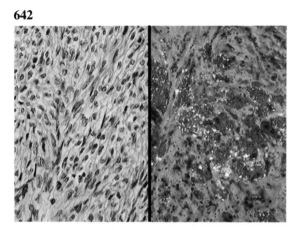

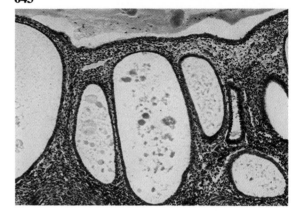

642 **Thecoma of the ovary** (8470) Same lesion as in **641**. Section showing interlacing bundles of spindle and polyhedral cells with rather pale almost clear cytoplasm. On the right cryostat section stained with scarlet red and viewed with polarised light, showing sudanophilic birefringent lipid in the cytoplasm. *(H&E × 83) (Scarlet red polarised × 83)*

643 **Cystic hyperplasia of the endometrium** (8600) from a case shown in **641** and **642**. *(H&E × 13)*

644 **Granulosa-cell tumour (carcinoma)** (8623) from a 47-year-old woman with a history of irregular menstruation over the past two years. A large (23 × 18 × 12 cm) solid tumour replaced the right ovary, the left appeared normal and the endometrium was hyperplastic and cystic. The cut surface of the tumour shows very characteristic pale-white trabeculae with small clefts bounded by white and yellow solid neoplasm and brown to red areas of haemorrhage and necrosis. There is a peripheral rim of connective tissue and the serosa shows no involvement. Histologically the sections showed follicular, microcystic and cylindromatous areas with mitoses up to 3 per HP field.

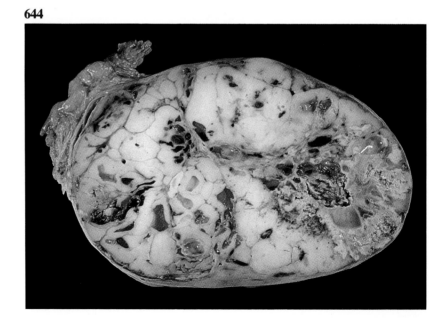
644

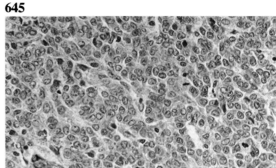

645 Granulosa-cell tumour (8623) Section of a lesion shown in **644** illustrating the uniformity of nuclei, trabecular arrangement and mitotic activity. *(H&E × 133)*

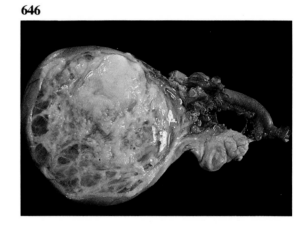

646 Leiomyoma (8600) of broad ligament from a 41-year-old woman with a 10cm in diameter swelling alongside the ovary. Frozen section was reported as showing degenerative changes in a fibroleiomyoma. No evidence of malignancy was seen in the paraffin sections.

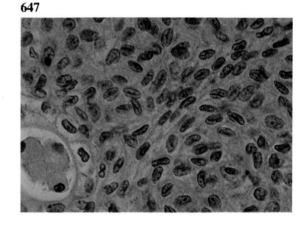

647 Brenner tumour of the ovary (9000) from a 41-year-old woman with an in situ carcinoma of the cervix treated by hysterectomy. The right ovary contained a 1cm hard nodule, which on section shows the typical histological appearance of a simple Brenner tumour with characteristic 'grooved' nuclei. It is not uncommon to find Brenner tumours contained within a pseudomucinous cystadenoma. *(H&E × 330)*

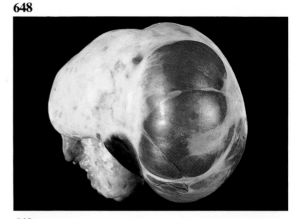

648

648 Adenofibroma of the ovary (9010) from a 33-year-old woman who complained of abdominal pain. The left ovary was enlarged (12 × 12 × 9cm) with smooth outer surface, white and opaque over nearly one half which is solid and with white whorled fibromatous cut surface, transparent and glistening over the other half which is cystic, with clear watery fluid filling the smooth lined spaces. Sections were reported as showing appearances of cystic adenofibroma.

649

649 Dermoid cyst of the ovary (9080) from a 62-year-old spinster who complained of intermittent abdominal pain and distension for six months. At laparotomy a right ovarian cystic mass (11 × 9 × 9cm) was partially torsed. The wall is generally thin and the contents include sebaceous material and hair. *No* evidence of malignancy is seen.

650

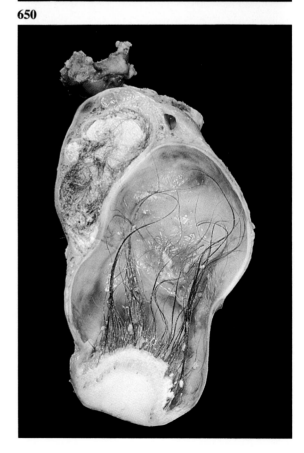

650 Dermoid cyst of both ovaries (9080) from a 29-year-old woman requesting sterilisation. Both ovaries showed dermoid cysts the larger (9 × 5 × 4.5cm) showing two main loculi each filled with sebaceous material and hair, seen to arise from a mamilla towards one end. The other was 7 × 5 × 4cm and showed a similar appearance.

651

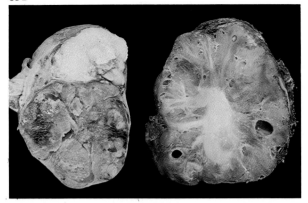

652

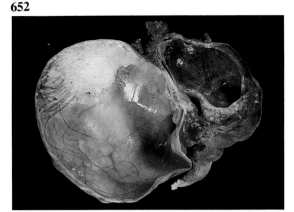

651 Struma ovarii (9090) On the left the ovary from a 65-year-old woman with post-menopausal bleeding and found to have adenoacanthoma of the uterus. The ovary is enlarged (6×5×4cm) and its cut surface shows a cystic part and a larger solid light-brown part with naked eye appearance of colloid rich thyroid tissue which it is histologically. On the right a struma ovarii showing malignant histological characteristics from a patient with thyrotoxicosis, which resolved after excision of the ovarian tumour.

653 Dermoid cyst (9080) containing teeth. (Same lesion as in **652**.)

652 Dermoid cyst (9080) containing teeth from a 31-year-old woman with tubal ectopic pregnancy. The 12cm long fallopian tube contains a 4 × 2.5cm gestation sac. The cyst is 6cm in diameter with 4cm wide ridge from which grow hairs and teeth (see **653**).

653

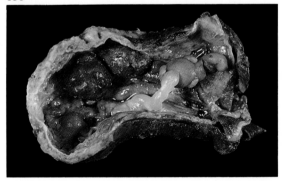

654

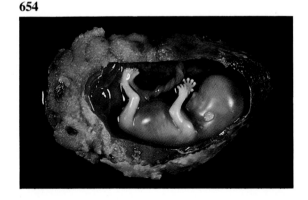

655

Placenta (T88)

654 Uterine abortion (normal foetus) (2630) from a 25-year-old woman Para 2/1, nine weeks since last menstrual period. The specimen is a complete conceptus in the form of a pyriform mass (10×6×4.5cm) with 6cm in diameter placenta and apparently normal 5cm (CR) foetus. The cause for the abortion was not apparent from study of the sections of the placenta and foetus.

655 Uterine abortion (abnormal foetus) (2630) from a 22-year-old primigravida. There was 10 weeks amenorrhoea, then spontaneous abortion of an intact gestation sac (6×3cm) with thin placenta overall. The foetus 1.6cm long, has an unduly small head and limbs, and the cord is a mere 1.4cm long. Five dark-red ovoid (6–12mm) swellings in the placenta are areas of intervillous thrombosis; chorionic villi showed degeneration, fibrosis and focal calcification.

656

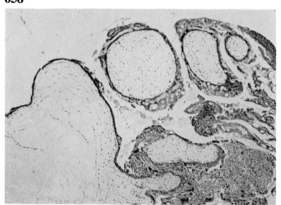

657

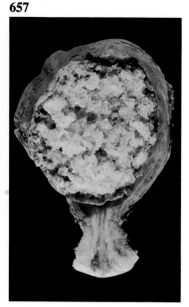

656 Early implanted ovum (2630) found by chance in the endometrial curettings from a 27-year-old woman who complained of menorrhagia. The endometrium showed decidual change and the implanted ovum was 2 mm in diameter, estimated age 17 days. *(H&E × 13)*

657 Hydatidiform mole (9100) from a 31-year-old woman with vaginal discharge, bleeding and uterus large for dates. The specimen is a large (14 × 11 × 10 cm) uterus occupied by a mass of hydatidiform villi up to 12 mm in diameter. There is only minimal erosion of myometrium.

658

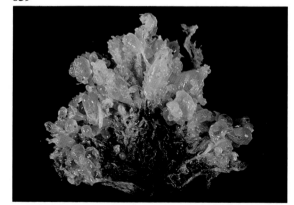

659

658 Hydatidiform mole (9100) Section of hydatidiform villi to show liquefaction centrally, avascularity and trophoblastic overgrowth. *(H&E × 13)*

659 Partial hydatidiform mole (9100) from a woman with four months amenorrhoea but uterus not enlarging, and no quickening. An oval mass (6 × 3 × 2 cm) of manifestly hydatidiform vesicular (up to 10 mm) tissue towards one end and more normal looking placental tissue at the other but without recognisable foetus.

9 Endocrine glands

660

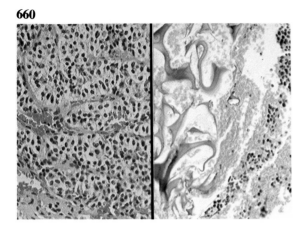

661

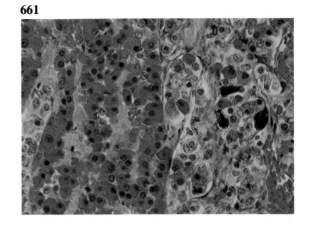

662

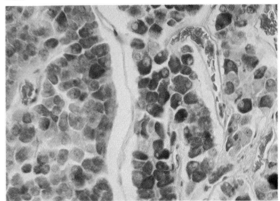

Pituitary gland (T00)

660 Chromophobe adenoma of the pituitary gland (8270) from a 65-year-old woman with bitemporal hemianopia and panhypopituitarism. A solid tumour was found compressing the chiasma and removal was attempted. Eight pieces (up to 5mm) were received and sections show appearances of chromophobe adenoma. Three months later recurrence of symptoms led to re-exploration. Small pieces of residual adenoma and pieces of gelfoam were received and are shown in the section stained with OFG in which eosinophil cells stain yellow and basophil cells stain purple. *(H&E × 83, OFG × 53)*

661 Eosinophil adenoma of the pituitary gland (8280) from a 45-year-old woman with acromegaly. Section stained with Biggart's eosin isamine blue shows eosinophils red, basophils blue-purple, and chromophobes a pale grey or unstained. *(Eosin Isamine blue × 133)*

662 Basophil adenoma of the pituitary gland (8300) from a 58-year-old hypertensive obese woman, clinically regarded as having Cushing's syndrome. *(Eosin Isamine blue × 133)*

663

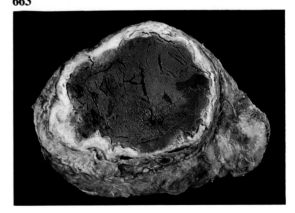

Adrenal gland (T93)

663 Calcified adenoma of the right adrenal gland (8370) from a woman with chronic cholecystitis. The lesion was recognised on the cholecystogram and excised at the time of cholecystectomy. It is a (9 × 6.5 × 4cm) gland containing a (7 × 5.5 × 4cm) heavily calcified mass which can only be cut with difficulty using a diamond saw. The whole specimen weighs 95 g. Sections showed cholesterol-containing material in the centre, an irregular partly calcified partly ossified shell 2mm to 5mm thick and here and there recognisable adenoma composed of eosinophil polyhedral cells.

664 **Cortical adenoma (brown tumour) of the adrenal gland** (8370) from a 49-year-old man with Cushing's syndrome with hypertension, osteoporosis with fractured ribs, generalised weakness and moon face. Cortisol levels showed no diurnal variation or betamethasone suppression. IVP showed right adrenal mass. At operation, right adrenal gland contained a 3cm spherical tumour. The adrenal cortex appeared thin and atrophic while the adenoma had a dark-brown and yellow cut surface. Histologically the lesion was reported as cortical adenoma with varied cell content. Some areas show large cells with pale staining finely granular cytoplasm rich in sudanophilic lipid; others show large cells with abundant brown pigment granules in densely eosinophilic cytoplasm, while other areas comprise small cells compactly arranged. Mitoses are exceptionally rare, though there are some bizarre large nuclei. Chrome fixation produced no chromaffin reaction.

665 **Cortical adenoma (brown tumour) of the adrenal gland** (8370) in Cushing's syndrome. Section of the lesion in **664** showing the three types of cell in Giemsa stained section. (Giemsa's stain is useful in demonstrating the granules in phaeochromocytoma after chrome fixation.) *(×330)*

666 **Phaeochromocytoma of the left adrenal gland** (8700) from a 37-year-old man with paroxysmal hypertensive episodes. A mass was demonstrated radiologically, and there were raised levels of catecholamines. At operation the enlarged left adrenal gland with 4.5cm in diameter light-brown coloured tumour (phaeo in Greek means dun-coloured) was removed. Histologically it was a typical phaeochromocytoma.

667 **Phaeochromocytoma** (8700) Same lesion as in **666**. Section to show alveolar arrangement of polyhedral cells resembling those of normal medulla – they have abundant eosinophilic cytoplasm, with fine pigment granules giving a positive reaction after chrome fixation. Mitoses are usually quite rare and most phaeochromocytomas are benign. *(H&E×83)*

664

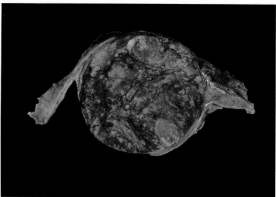

665

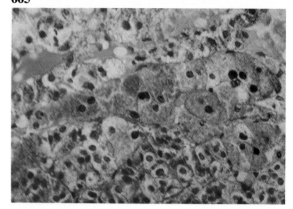

666

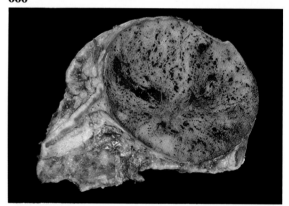

667

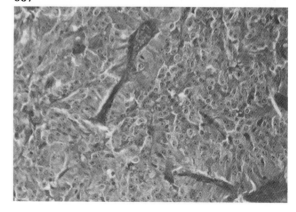

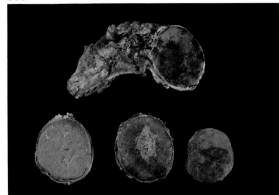

668 Multiple phaeochromocytomas (8700) One adrenal gland and three accessory chromaffin organs of Zuckerkandl contained tumours each about 3cm in diameter, and another tumour was so intimately connected to large vessels that it could not be removed.

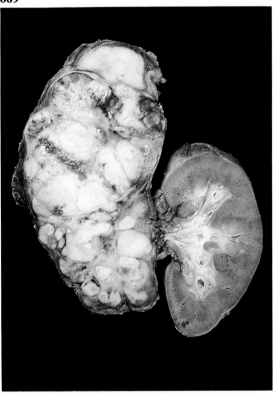

669 Neuroblastoma (ganglioneuroblastoma) (9493) of the left gland from a six-year-old boy with recurrent abdominal pain and palpable mass in the left hypochondrium, with raised blood levels of catecholamines. At operation a large ($12 \times 6 \times 5$cm) neoplasm lay alongside the left kidney, completely replacing the left adrenal gland. The cut surface was white and nodular with yellow areas of necrosis and gritty calcified nodules. Histologically initial sections showed appearances of neuroblastoma, but additional sections showed differentiation with ganglion cell formation.

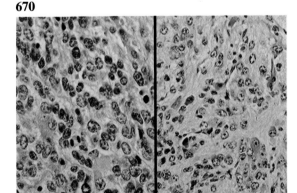

670 Ganglioneuroblastoma (9493) Same lesion as in **669**. Section shows (on left) sheets of darkly staining cells with abundant fibrillary stroma and with mitotic activity, on the right ganglion cell formation. (*H&E $\times 83$, $\times 53$*)

Carotid body (T94)

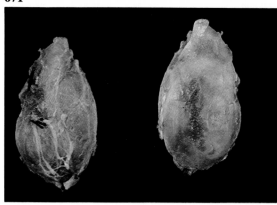

671 **Carotid body tumour** (8690) from the neck of a young woman. It is a pyriform mass (3.5×2×2cm) with smooth outer surface and solid pale-pink to buff cut surface with scattered dark-red areas. Cryostat section was reported as showing unusually pleomorphic polyhedral cells, arranged in sheets and clusters around thin-walled vessels in keeping with chemodectoma (carotid body tumour).

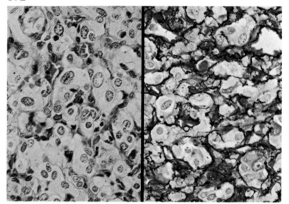

672 **Carotid body tumour** (8690) Section of a lesion shown in **671**. On the left H&E section shows typical 'Zellballen' of chemodectoma. On the right reticulin stain outlining these alveolar masses. Electron-micrography confirmed the diagnosis in demonstrating neurosecretory granules in the cytoplasm of the cells. *(×133)*

Thyroid gland (T96)

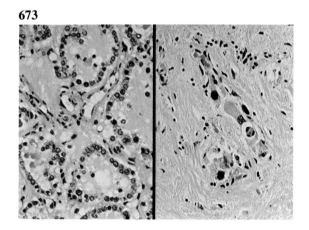

673 **Post-irradiation changes in the thyroid gland** (1130) after treatment with radioactive iodine. On the left section showing early changes, including scanty colloid, irregularly swollen darkly staining endothelial and epithelial cell nuclei in varying stages of degeneration. On the right section shows late changes with replacement fibrosis, bizarre giant nuclei (epithelial, endothelial, and histiocytic), and sparse lymphocytic infiltrate. *(H&E×83)*

674

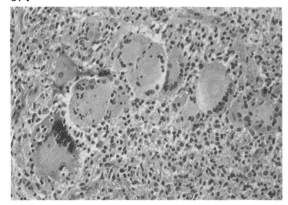

674 Giant-cell thyroiditis (subacute thyroiditis of de Quervain) (7233) Cryostat section of a biopsy from a recently painful swollen thyroid gland of a young woman showing multinucleate phagocytes ingesting released colloid, and mixed leucocytic infiltrate. *(×53)*

675

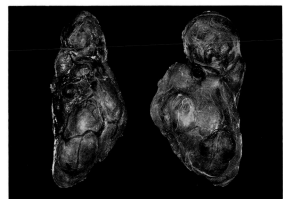

675 Colloid nodular goitre (7233) from a 46-year-old woman with a history of large goitre for many years. A total of 366 g of tissue was removed in the form of two lobes each 12.5 cm long and 5.5 cm broad.

676 Colloid nodular goitre (7233) Same lesion as shown in **675**. The cut surface shows marked nodularity, with areas of calcification, degeneration, fibrosis and cyst formation and histological sections showed appearances of benign nodular colloid goitre.

676

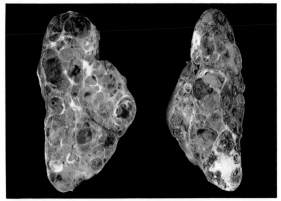

677

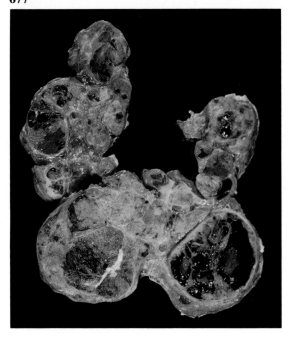

677 Nodular colloid goitre (7233) from a 61-year-old man with a three-year history of enlarging non-toxic huge goitre. The specimen weighs 545 g and consists of two portions (13×11×8 cm and 10×5.5×4.5 cm respectively). The whole gland is grossly distorted by more than 45 large nodules up to 5 cm in diameter. There are many areas of degeneration haemorrhage, fibrosis and calcification. No evidence of malignancy was seen in the many sections examined.

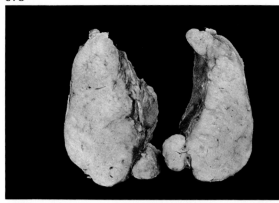

678 Diffuse thyroid hyperplasia (thyrotoxicosis) (7300) from a 39-year-old woman with a goitre and clinical thyrotoxicosis for six months. Subtotal thyroidectomy removed 40g of tissue in the form of two lobes, each with meaty pale uniform cut surface. Histological sections showed tall columnar epithelial cells lining vesicles deficient in colloid, which show vacuoles at the periphery and with some lymphoid follicular hyperplasia.

679

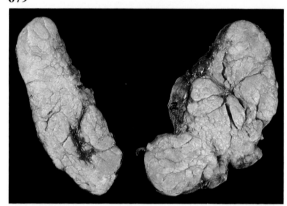

679 Hashimoto's thyroiditis (autoimmune diffuse thyroiditis) (7661) from a hypothyroid patient with a very large goitre and very high blood level of thyroid antibodies. The gland weighed 400g and its cut surface is pale and trabeculated.

680

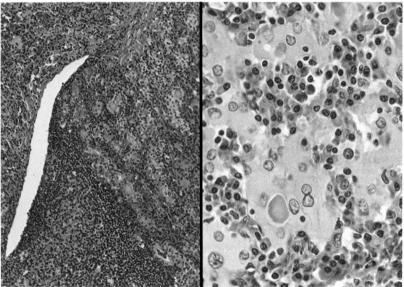

680 Hashimoto's thyroiditis (7661) Same lesion as in **679**. Section shows replacement of thyroid tissue by masses of round cells including many plasma cells: remaining thyroid epithelium sometimes appears brightly eosinophilic – Askanazy cell change. Lymphoid follicles with germinal centres and lymphatic clefts in the fibrous septae make up a pathognomonic histological picture. *(H&E × 33, × 133)*

681

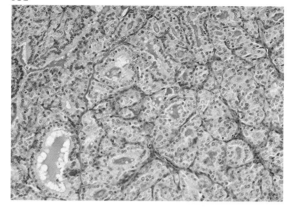

681 Diffuse thyroid hyperplasia (7300) Section to show columnar cell proliferation (mitoses were easy to find in the section), scanty pale staining colloid with artefactual vacuolation seen bottom left. Only a few areas showed lymphoid infiltration and follicles with germinal centres. *(H&E × 53)*

682

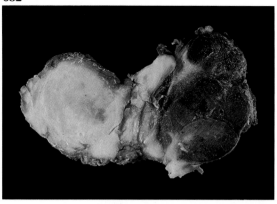

682 'Riedel's thyroiditis' (7662) from a woman who complained of hoarseness with dysphagia for several months. There was a large goitre and at operation it felt rubbery and appeared pale. Extensions of the mass infiltrated the neck muscles and passed down behind the sternum. The specimen is a 32 g mass comprising a near normal (4 × 2.5 cm) left lobe and firm pale right lobe (3 × 3 cm) and isthmus. On initial histological examination the extensive fibrosis associated with large aggregates of round cells (lymphocytes and plasma cells with some histiocytes) was thought compatible with the diagnosis of Riedel's thyroiditis, but concern was expressed that the lesion might have a lymphomatous basis. The patient died within a short while. The necropsy diagnosis was malignant lymphoma.

683

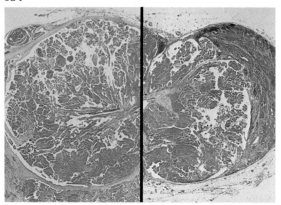

683 Papillary carcinoma of the thyroid gland (8053) with metastases in ipselateral lymph nodes in a 17-year-old boy.

684

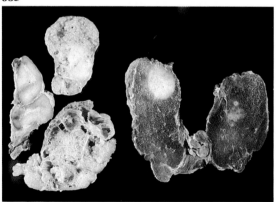

684 Papillary carcinoma of the thyroid gland (8053) from a 64-year-old woman who complained of a choking sensation and swelling in the neck for six years. A hard fixed (10 × 6 × 5 cm) mass weighing 106 g with enlarged nodes was removed at operation. The cut surface was uniformly papilliform, gritty in parts; histologically sections showed papillary carcinoma with calcispherites and lymphatic permeation in the adjacent connective tissues. The nodes showed almost total replacement by metastases showing similar papillary pattern. Section on left shows thyroid lesion, on right lymph node metastasis. *(H&E × 3.5, × 4)*

685

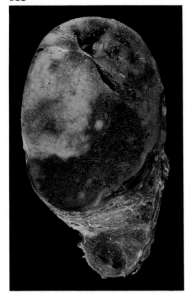

686

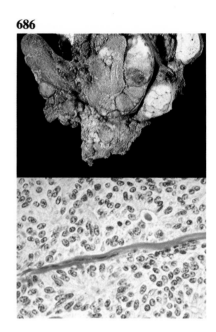

685 Adenoma ?adenocarcinoma (8142) from a 46-year-old woman with a five-year history of an enlarged thyroid gland. The specimen is an enlarged lobe (10 × 8 × 5 cm) containing an ovoid well-circumscribed fleshy mass (8 × 7 × 5 cm). The cut surface shows haemorrhagic areas and the surrounding thyroid tissue is compressed: there are two smaller nodules towards the upper pole. Cryostat section caused difficulty and

was reported as atypical acidophil adenoma showing cytological features of malignancy in that there were bizarre large nuclei and mitotic activity with abnormal forms: final diagnosis to await paraffin sections. These in fact appeared to confirm that the lesion was well circumscribed, did not show any vascular invasion, and did not warrant further immediate treatment.

686 Cellular follicular adenoma ?follicular adeno-carcinoma (8142) from a 17-year-old boy. Section shows follicular pattern and a cell in mitosis. Seventeen years later the patient returned with extreme dyspnoea caused by a huge goitre, and with numerous enlarged nodes on both sides of the neck but mainly on the ipselateral (right) side. The sections of this lesion were quite like those of the original lesion, though overtly invasive. He survived for a short time after the thyroidectomy. *(H&E × 83)*

687

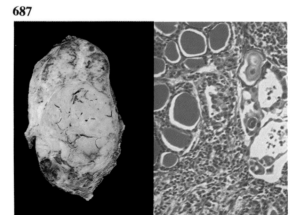

688

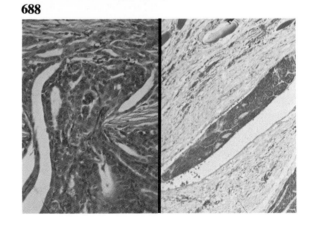

687 Follicular adenocarcinoma of the thyroid gland (8143) from a 75-year-old man who complained of swelling and pain in the region of the thyroid for 1 year. The mass of thyroid tissue (9 × 6 × 4.5 cm) has an irregular nodular surface and towards one end there is a pale fleshy mass (5 × 4 × 4 cm), while the rest of the gland has a mottled yellow-and-grey appearance with scattered haemorrhages. Sections showed well-differentiated follicular carcinoma infiltrating adjacent thyroid and with vascular invasion in several blocks; on the right, section of well-differentiated adenocarcinoma showing calcispherites. *(H&E × 53)*

688 Adenocarcinoma of the thyroid (8143) in a young policewoman. Section to show, on left, invasive break-through capsule and, on right, carcinomatous tissue within lumen of vein. *(H&E × 83, × 13)*

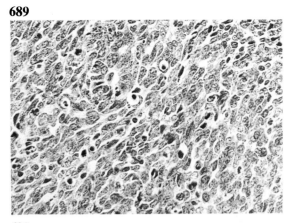

689

689   Anaplastic carcinoma of the thyroid (8233) from a 48-year-old woman with a goitre and enlarged cervical lymph nodes. Section was reported as showing anaplastic, in places spindle-cell carcinoma. *(H&E × 83)*

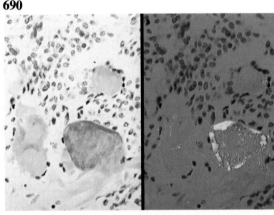

690

690   Medullary carcinoma of the thyroid (8233) with amyloid stroma from a 49-year-old woman with swelling in the neck and pyrexia, initially diagnosed as having papillary adenocarcinoma with collagenous stroma. Eight years later she presented with diarrhoea. The physician requested review of the sections when the correct diagnosis became apparent. Section stained with congo red demonstrates amyloid in the stroma; viewed with polarised light it exhibits dichroic birefringence. This is now regarded as a tumour of parafollicular cells (C-cells) and is known genetically to be associated with phaeochromocytoma and other endocrine diseases. *(Congo red × 53)*

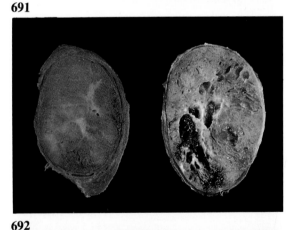

691

691   Adenoma of the thyroid gland (8350) on the left from a 62-year-old euthyroid woman with a swelling in the right side of the neck. A large (6 × 4 × 3.5 cm) ovoid mass weighing 38 g consists of an adenoma with a narrow rim of compressed atrophic thyroid tissue. Histologically it was a benign follicular colloid-rich adenoma. On the right from a thyrotoxic young man with a lump in the neck. An (5 × 4 × 3 cm) adenoma, pale-brown and fleshy at the periphery but with central areas of fibrosis, haemorrhage and cystic change. Sections showed follicular adenoma with great variation in epithelial height, in places showing papillary folds, the appearance being consistent with a hyperfunctioning state.

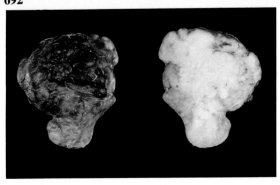

692

692   Malignant lymphoma of the thyroid gland (probable T-cell tumour – struma reticulosa) (9593) from a 73-year-old woman with asymptomatic swelling in the neck noted by her GP. The specimen is 8 × 7 × 4.5 cm and the cut surface shows white nodular neoplasm replacing rather pale-brown thyroid tissue. Sections showed diffuse infiltration of the thyroid by malignant lymphoma, the cells ranging from small lymphocytes to large reticulum cells and showing considerable mitotic activity. The remaining thyroid tissue shows appearances of a chronic thyroiditis of the autoimmune type.

Parathyroid glands (T97)

693   Diffuse hyperplasia of all four parathyroid glands
(7300) from a 28-year-old man with acute hyper-
calcaemic crisis: emergency parathyroidectomy at
midnight produced enlarged (up to 14mm long) glands
all showing hyperplasia with remarkable mitotic activity
(up to 7 mitoses in a HP field). *(H&E × 33)*

693

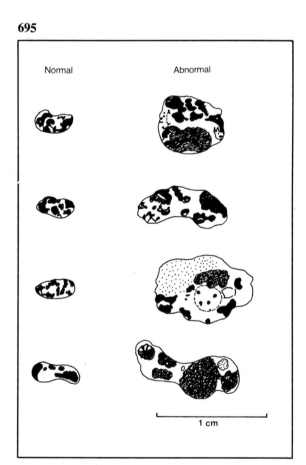

694

695

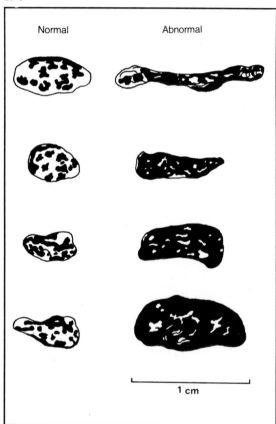

694   Diffuse hyperplasia of the parathyroid glands
(7300) Same case as in **693**. Line drawing to show
shape and size of affected glands alongside normal
control.

**695   'Nodular hyperplasia' of all four parathyroid
glands** (7300) from a 49-year-old woman. All four
glands showed abnormal nodules of varying structure
and neither on cryostat nor paraffin section was it
possible to be certain that the process was nodular
hyperplasia or adenomatosis (pluriglandular syndrome).
The answer was forthcoming four years later when an
insulinoma (see **703**) was removed from the pancreas.
Line drawing to show shape and size of affected glands
alongside normal control. The largest gland measured
$10 \times 6 \times 6$mm.

696 Adenoma of the parathyroid gland (8140) from a 44-year-old man with a long history of renal stone and intermittent hypercalcaemia. A mass was removed from the right side and it contained a brown tumour (2 × 1.2 × 1 cm) which on cryostat section was composed mainly of chief cells, with pale cytoplasm though with some areas of more deeply eosinophil cells. Section is shown on the right. *(H&E × 53)*

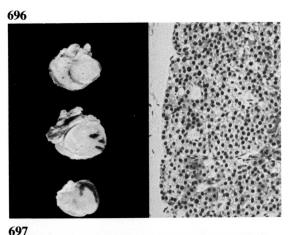

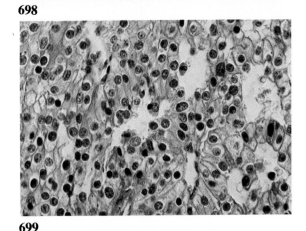

697 Nodular hyperplasia (adenomatosis) of the parathyroid glands (8140) in a 31-year-old man on renal dialysis for chronic renal failure and regarded clinically as manifesting tertiary hyperparathyroidism. The glands ranged in size from 10 mm to 25 mm in diameter and all show brown cut surfaces with paler nodules. Histologically the nodular appearance is made up of chief cells among which there are nodules of oxyphil cells of varying size. In some areas there is acinar formation with colloid-like content in the lumens.

698 Carcinoma of the parathyroid gland (8143) from a 54-year-old woman with a tragic history of an above-knee amputation of the left leg when aged 43 for non-union of fracture; nine years later pathological fracture of the right femur and then 'cysts' of the long bones. A biopsy of a cyst of the tibia showed appearances of osteitis fibrosa cystica: an exploration of a swelling in the neck revealed a neoplasm of the parathyroid with features suggesting carcinoma rather than adenoma. Four months later excision of an undoubted carcinoma, in several pieces, in all weighing about 10 g, was attempted but the patient died the following day. At necropsy the skull and most of the bones were elastic. There were metastatic nodules of carcinoma infiltrating the oesophagus and paratracheal tissues. Section shows solid cellular masses of polyhedral cells (chief cells) with variation in nuclear size and occasional mitosis. *(H&E × 133)*

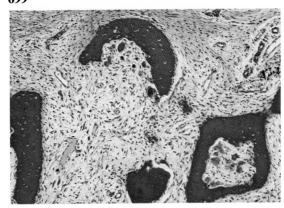

699 Osteitis fibrosa cystica (7644) Section of a lesion of the tibia from the same case as in **698** showing fibrosis, Howship's lacunae with osteoclasts and scattered siderophages: undecalcified sections showed widened osteoid seams. *(Red & yellow × 33)*

Thymus (T98)

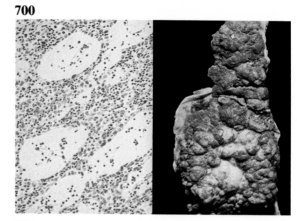

700 Thymoma (8583) Section of a spherical mass removed from the thymus of a 37-year-old woman with myasthenia gravis. The lesions on the left consisted of small lymphocyte-like cells and larger pale staining epithelial cells in lobular and trabecular arrangement with cystic areas. There was much infiltration of adjacent thymus tissues with spread into mediastinal fat. A muscle biopsy showed lymphorrhages and marrow was hypoplastic. The patient died years later with recurrence of the lesion in the left pleural cavity, shown on right. *(H&E × 33)*

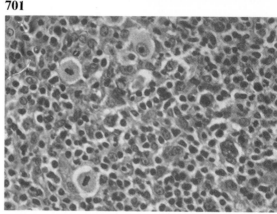

701 Thymoma (Hodgkin type) (8583) Section of a large mass replacing the thymus in a young woman. Histologically the lesion was indistinguishable from Hodgkin's disease. *(H&E × 133)*

Islets of Langerhans (T99)

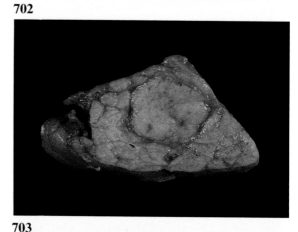

702 Insulinoma (islet cell tumour) (8150) from a woman with hypoglycaemia: at laparotomy a (12 × 11 × 10mm) nodule could just be felt close to the plane of excision. The cut surface was gritty. It was reported on cryostat section as an islet-cell tumour, with striking acinar pattern and numerous calcispherites. Electron-microscopy confirmed the diagnosis.

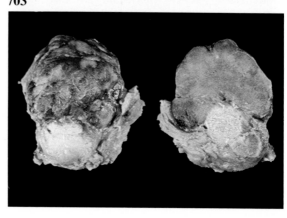

703 Islet-cell tumour (8150) from a 49-year-old woman who four years before had nodular hyperplasia of all four parathyroid glands (**695**). On left the external surface appears nodular; on right the cut surface shows pale calcified areas. Histologically this lesion was reported as an apudoma of islet-cell type.

10 Nervous system, eyes and ears

Meninges (TX1)

704 Meningioma of the left parietal region (9530) from a 76-year-old woman with signs of a left cortical lesion and a swelling of the skull. A flap of dura (6 × 5 cm) with a solid mass (5 × 4 × 2 cm) apparently penetrating it, and a piece of skull (7.5 × 6 cm) bearing an ovoid plaque on its outer surface. The sections showed that the meningioma had infiltrated marrow spaces leading to expansion of the haversian canals but in general without destroying much bone.

704

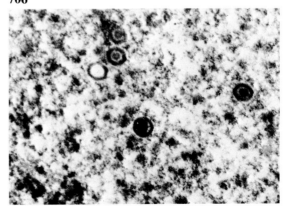

705

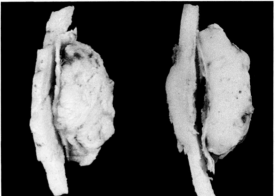

706

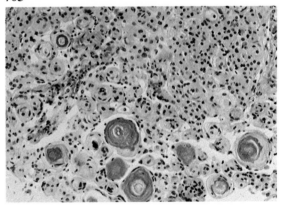

705 Meningioma from the foramen magnum (9530) of a 60-year-old woman with a five-year history of increasing spastic quadriplegia. The lesion was removed piecemeal and section shows appearance of meningioma with psammoma bodies. In cryostat sections there is often difficulty in distinguishing meningioma from chemodectoma, neurilemmoma and neurofibroma: but the alkaline phosphatase content of meningioma is often high while in the others it is low or absent. *(H&E × 53)*

Cerebrum (TX2)

706 Herpes encephalitis (4000) Virus demonstrated electronmicrographically in a biopsy of temporal lobe from a patient with herpetic encephalitis. *(× 65,000)*

707 **Gemistocytic astrocytoma** (9413) from the right pole of a 51-year-old woman with progressive confusion, epilepsy and left hemiparesis. Section shows distinctive large globoid cells with coarse fibrillary processes. A significant proportion of gemistocytic astrocytomas progress to anaplastic astrocytoma. *(Modified H&E × 133)*

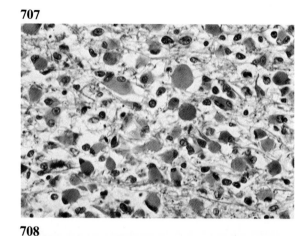

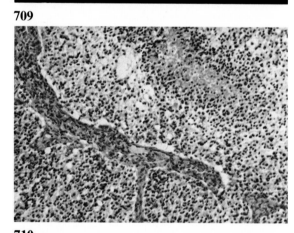

708 **Anaplastic astrocytoma (Grade IV)** (9443) from the left frontal pole of a 50-year-old man with a short history of headache and vomiting and found to have gross papilloedema. The specimen is part of the frontal lobe, measures 6 × 5 × 3 cm and includes a haemorrhagic necrotic neoplasm (3 × 2 × 5 cm).

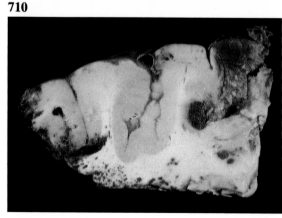

709 **Grade IV astrocytoma** (9443) Section of a lesion shown in **708** displaying high cellularity, mitoses, nuclear pleomorphism, necrosis, characteristic new vessel formation with endothelial proliferation. *(H&E × 53)*

710 **Oligodendroglioma from the left frontal lobe** (9453) of a 46-year-old chartered accountant with sudden onset of epilepsy, headache, lethargy and vomiting. CAT scan showed a frontal lobe tumour, which in the specimen is friable and gritty being centred on subcortical white matter in wide flat nodular gyri.

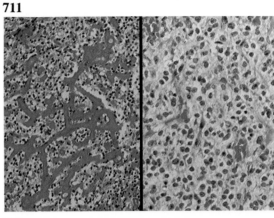

711

711   Oligodendroglioma (9453) Same case as in **710**.
The histological sections show typical box-like cells and
accompanying calcification. Mitoses were numerous in
some areas. *(H&E×53, ×83)*

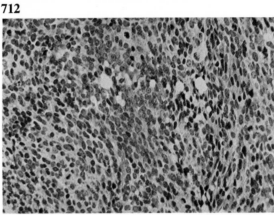

712

Cerebellum (TX5)

712   Medulloblastoma from posterior fossa (9473) of an
eight-year-old girl. Section was reported as showing
embryonal type neuroepithelium but with occasional
large ganglion cells. *(H&E×133)*

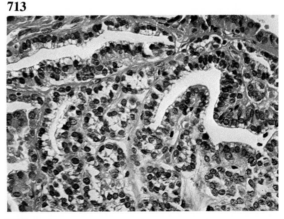

713

Spinal cord (TX7)

713   Ependymoma of the spinal cord (9391) from a
two-year-old boy with signs of spinal-cord compression.
Cryostat section was reported as showing papillary
ependymoma without pleomorphism, endothelial
proliferation or necrosis. *(H&E×133)*

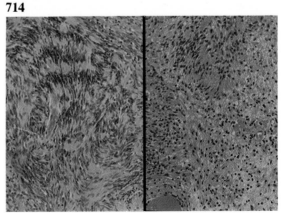

714

714   Neurilemmoma of the trigeminal nerve (9560) of a
34-year-old theatre assistant with a three-month history
of right side facial pain, diplopia and headache. The
specimen consisted of 30 pieces (up to 1.5cm in
diameter) of pale nodular neoplasm, histologically
showing on left typical Antoni type-A structure and on
right type-B structure. *(H&E×53)*

Eyes (TXX)

715 Chlamydial conjunctivitis (4000) from a service-man with severe bilateral conjunctivitis not responding to conventional treatment. The smear was made by lightly stroking the palpebral conjunctiva with the blunt end of a scalpel blade, then smearing the cells on a glass slide and staining it with Giemsa's stain. The intracytoplasmic Chlamydia are seen as a crescentic mass of tiny particles in the conjunctival epithelial cells. On the right **Molluscum contagiosum** (7347) bodies from a smear of lesions on the eyelids of a ten-year-old girl: they stain strongly with phloxine. *(Giemsa × 330), phloxine × 53)*

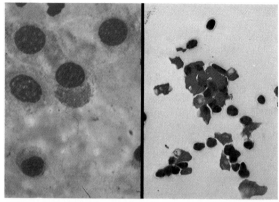

716 Corneal abscess (4173) with perforation (suppurative keratitis) from a 69-year-old hospital porter with hypopyon, corneal ulcer and triradiate rupture of the inflamed cornea. On the right a **detached retina** (3324) in aphakic eye from a 43-year-old man, who had been blind for 12 years. The eye became painful and was removed. The specimen shows total retinal detachment and cyst formation.

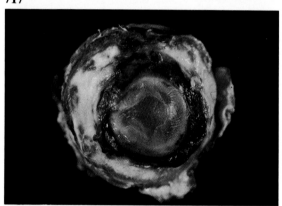

717 Post-herpes zoster anaesthesia (4303) with corneal ulcer in an 80-year-old woman who developed Pseudomonas endophthalmitis requiring exenteration. The corneal ulcer is 8 × 5 mm.

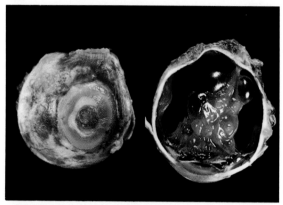

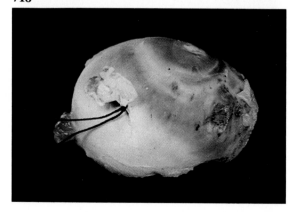

718 Staphyloma of the left eye (4544) from a 54-year-old woman who was blind since childhood. The eye became painful and was enucleated.

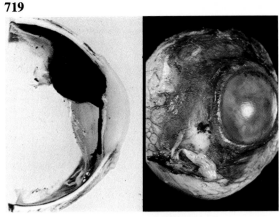

719 **Malignant melanoma of the ciliary body** (8723) on the nasal aspect over its outer third; the iris appears black as a result of a melanoma affecting one-fifth of the circumference. The pupil is irregular. The sclera adjacent to the lesion shows three small (two are pinpoint and the other just measurable at $2 \times 1\,mm$) areas of brown pigmentation lying a few millimetres wide of the corneoscleral junction.

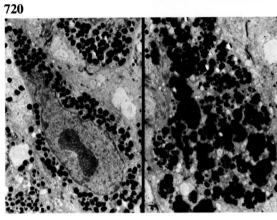

720 **Malignant melanoma** (8723) Electronmicroscopy of the largest area (see **719**) confirmed that it consisted of neoplastic melanocytes (on left) and melanophages (on right). *(× 4,500)*

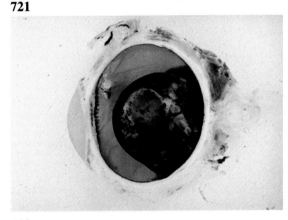

721 **Choroidal malignant melanoma** (8723) from a 76-year-old woman with deteriorating vision in the left eye. A large (2 cm) deeply pigmented tumour is present posteromedially close to the optic disc, and there was extensive retinal detachment. Sections showed a varied histological pattern with polyhedral large cells and spindle cells, abundant melanin and moderate mitotic activity. There was only superficial invasion of sclera and no demonstrable extension outside the globe.

Ears (TXY)

722 **Aural polyp from the left external auditory meatus** (4300) from a 52-year-old man with a long history of chronic otitis media and discharging ear. The $(17 \times 6 \times 5\,mm)$ polyp showed vascular oedematous stroma densely packed with plasma cells and lymphocytes as well as neutrophil polymorphonuclear leukocytes and macrophages and was covered by an epithelium consisting of stratified columnar and squamous cells. Numerous Russell bodies – densely eosinophilic spherules of varied size – are present in the areas where the plasma cells predominate, and are shown in a section stained with phloxine haematoxylin lissamine flavine. *(Phloxine HLF × 133)*

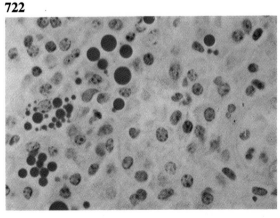

723 **Tympanosclerosis from the right ear** (4801) of a 37-year-old woman with progressive deafness since 16 years of age. At operation tympanosclerotic plaques were present on the membrana tympanum and on the ossicles. Stapedectomy and prosthetic replacement was carried out. The specimen shows the stirrup-shaped piece of bone mainly of lamellar type, with cartilaginous areas on the footplate and both crura covered with collagenous, poorly cellular fibrous tissue. *(van Gieson ×5)*

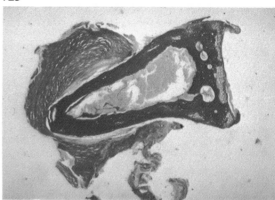

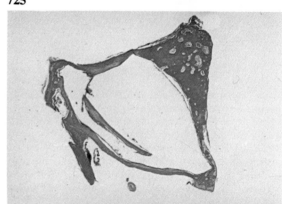

724 **Otosclerosis** (4801) Stapedectomy from a 44-year-old woman with progressive deafness. The stapes shows thickening and opacity of the footplate which histologically shows the typical pagetoid appearance of otosclerosis. *(×6)*

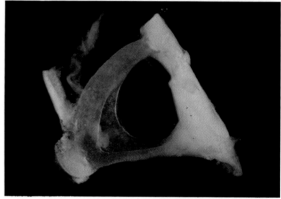

725 **Otosclerosis** (4801) Same case as in **724**. Section of the whole specimen showing the abnormal thickened footplate. *(×6)*

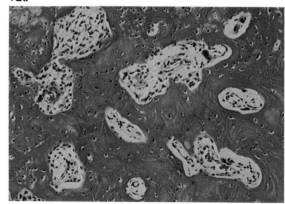

726 **Otosclerosis** (4801) Same case as in **725**. Section on left showing enlarged haversian systems containing vascular fibroblastic tissue and with osteoblasts and osteoblastic activity: replacement of lamellar bone with fibrous woven bone in irregular blocks leads to the mosaic pattern of cement lines. *(H&E×53)*

In surgical pathology practice one often sees very large cells of dimensions which warrant the title 'giant cell': often an eponymous title has been given and examiners are prone to ask about them. Already in this Atlas we have illustrated giant cells in a variety of inflammatory, metabolic, and neoplastic disorders (see 16, 24, 29, 32, 35, 80, 97, 118, 165, 175, 188, 203, 206, 243, 259, 263, 281, 297, 302, 373, 393, 496, 497, 538, 541, 615, 623, 673, 674 and 699). The following illustrations show further examples of lesions characterised by giant-cell formation, with eponymous designations where applicable.

727

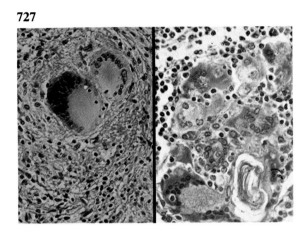

727 Langhans' type giant cell, on the left, in tuberculosis; on the right, **giant cells around a Schaumann body** in Boeck's sarcoidosis. *(×83) (×133)*

728

728 Asteroid in giant-cell in sarcoidosis on the left; on the right, **giant cell containing calcium oxalate in Crohn's disease.** *(×133) (×133)*

729

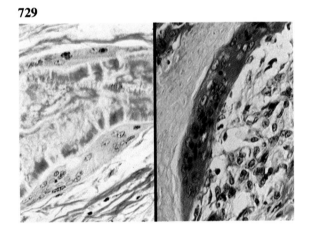

729 Amyloid deposit: on the left, giant cell surrounding an amyloid deposit. On the right, **giant cell of Malherbe** in pilomatrixoma. *(×133) (×133)*

730

730 Giant macrophage, on the left, **from a mucocoele of the vermiform appendix;** on the right, **Aschoff giant cell** in subendocardium of left atrial appendage. *(×53) (×133)*

731 **Touton giant cell in xanthoma,** on the left; on the right, **giant cell in Letterer-Siwe disease.** *(×133)* *(×133)*

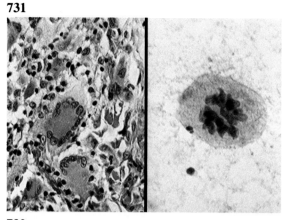

732 **Giant cell (osteoclast) with fibrinous mantle** in Von Recklinghausen's disease of the bone, on the left; on the right, **giant cell (osteoclast) in Paget's disease** of the bone. *(×53)* *(×133)*

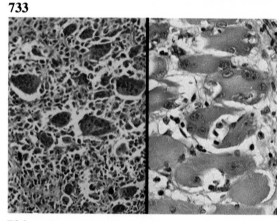

733 **Giant cell in giant-cell tumour of muscle,** on the left; on the right, **'muscle giant cell'** in traumatised vastus lateralis. *(×53)* *(×133)*

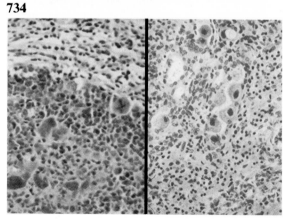

734 **Warthin-Finkeldey giant cell** in lymphoid tissue of vermiform appendix in measles, on the left; on the right, **renal tubule epithelial giant cells in cytomegalovirus infection.** *(×83)* *(×53)*

735

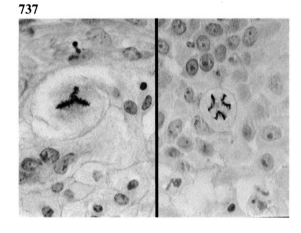

735 Physaliferous giant cells in chordoma, on the left; on the right, **giant cells in glioblastoma multiforme.** *(×133) (×83)*

736

736 Giant cell in malignant melanoma, on the left; on the right, giant cell in ascitic fluid from a woman with **squamous-cell carcinoma of the cervix uteri.** *(×83) (×133)*

737

737 Abnormal mitosis in a lipophage, on the left, on the surface of a vermiform appendix; on the right, **abnormal mitosis in oesophageal epithelium in oesophagitis.** *(×300) (×300)*

Note
Abnormal mitotic figures occasionally occur in non-malignant conditions. We have encountered them in several sites including proliferative phase endometrium, foci of endometriosis, in granulation tissue in the base of an amoebic ulcer of the skin, in renal tubular epithelium in distal tubule necrosis in a patient with extensive burns, in regenerating hepatocytes, and in reactive lymph nodes in pasteurellosis. On the other hand abnormal mitoses are a very common finding in highly malignant proliferating neoplasms, and are useful corroborative evidence in diagnosing malignancy.

Appendix

There is an ever increasing specialisation in pathological techniques today. Therefore it is becoming increasingly important for surgeons to think carefully before dropping a specimen straight into a jar of fixative.

Requirements of the microbiologist, electron-microscopist, histochemist, haematologist, cytologist, immunologist, pharmacologist and geneticist, as well as those of the histopathologist, have to be met if optimum results for the patient are to be achieved.

Unfixed uncontaminated material must be reserved for culture or animal inoculation. Fresh imprints are invaluable to the cytologist and haematologist. Tiny blocks, less than 1 mm cube, must be fixed immediately in special fixative preferably chilled (4°C) 3 per cent buffered gluteraldehyde, and sent to the laboratory in a refrigerated container or vacuum bucket if perfect electron-microscopic details are to be preserved. For accurate histochemical localisation of enzymes and avoidance of artefact, freezing in isopentane in liquid nitrogen (−180°C) has proven a satisfactory routine procedure. Pharmacological assays too may be possible on frozen tissue though some are best done on fresh tissue. Geneticists prefer fresh material. It is after consideration of such a battery of interested parties that the 'routine histology' has to be organised, and here there are further specialised techniques demanding particular processing and skills.

A knowledge of the common conditions allows one to establish routine schedules which work well whether the laboratory is close by or remote from the operating theatre. For example with swellings in the neck it is a matter of dividing the fresh specimen (a sharp cutting blade such as a dermatome is ideal): the smaller part goes to the microbiologist while the pathologist makes imprints, takes small pieces for cryostat section and for plastic embedding and routine blocks for processing to paraffin wax.

Importance of fresh specimens

Conveniently in a teaching department, receiving the fresh specimen enables photographs to be taken: the surgeon has both a legal and moral obligation to let the hospital pathologist have the complete unmutilated specimen on which to base his report – obviously if the pathologist receives only part of, or a very haphazardly slashed, specimen it is unlikely that his report will be accurate or reliable. Dividing specimens, then sending one piece to one pathologist and the other to another can only be condemned, because there is a grave risk of the patient getting the worst of two worlds rather than the best. Health and safety at work regulations are more strict today and excellent fixatives such as those containing Mercuric chloride are no longer used, although satisfactory substitutes have not been found.

For general fixation purposes buffered formalin seems at present to offer the best overall cover for preserving specimens and still allowing routine paraffin processing using automated processors to function satisfactorily and give a 24-hour service with small biopsies and a 48-hour service for large specimens. If material is required for publication or special teaching purposes it is essential to use special processing programmes, and cut sections of appropriate thickness, and stain them individually.

There is always urgency to human pathological specimens but in certain situations an 'urgent report' is required within 5 or 10 minutes and cryostat or frozen section can meet this demand. On the one hand when the surgeon is fully aware beforehand of the likely need for a cryostat section it should be possible to plan the timing of the operation to suit patient, surgeon, scientific officer and pathologist. On the other hand when the unexpected crops up and further treatment depends on the result, cryostat section of this can usually be arranged. However, it is as well to remember that there are certain situations where a rapid cryostat section cannot be expected to give a reasonable answer – for example in neoplasms where histological appearances are not the best guide to behaviour – or where it is not possible to cover the area without multiple blocks and sections, as in assessing whether or not there is residual neoplasm, or granulomatous lesions in the edges of resection of ileum in Crohn's disease. Cryostat section should not be sought if there is a known risk of tuberculosis or virus hepatitis.

Biopsies and processing

Skin

Skin biopsies taken with a scalpel are usually small, elliptical or wedge shaped with surfaces readily identifiable. One may embed the block in one piece, or as two (after a skew or longitudinal slice through any contained lesion), or in three by taking a middle transverse cut to include clearance at its minimum and two blocks at right angles towards the ends of the specimen. Punch biopsies may be difficult to orientate and require extra careful attention at blocking out. If fluorescent studies are required a piece should be taken for cryostat section, similarly if there is a likelihood of having to demonstrate lipid. Cysts are generally removed intact but it is often of value to aspirate a little of the contents for direct microscopy or chemical analysis. Wet preparations are ideal for identifying ciliated cells, spermatozoa in spermatocoele, squames and cholesterol crystals in branchial cleft cyst, pH testing verifies the presence of acid secretion in enterogenous cysts. Blocks of sebaceous or epidermal cysts process best if a middle cut is chosen. Calcific deposits can ruin microtome knives and it is useful to know that a specimen, if xrayed, contains calcium salts or bone. Lipid in xanthoma, histiocytoma, thecoma, liposarcoma, cholesterolosis of gallbladder, or in atheromatous arteries is best examined both as a cryostat and as paraffin sections; the cryostat section being cut in triplicate to have an unstained control for polarising microscopy, one for Sudan staining and one for H & E. Immunoperoxidase methods are now established for verifying cholesterol in sections. Lesions of nerve include stump neuroma, neurilemmoma or schwannoma and neurofibroma and demonstration of axis cylinders is useful in diagnosis. The Holmes Alcian A.V.19 method is a reliable one which works well on paraffin processed material.

Breast

Breast lesions are currently being assessed in many different ways in the various centres in UK. Cytological smears from small-bore needle aspiration in the hands of experts appears to be a useful adjunct to clinical and mammographic examination. Cryostat section is useful and reliable in breast lumps – however, there will always be an occasional lesion in which it is necessary to delay a decision on diagnosis until paraffin sections become available. Nipple discharges may be of various colours: it is always worthwhile examining a stained smear in case of intraduct carcinoma. Duct papilloma is easily missed if not searched for very carefully. Second tumours occur in breast sufficiently commonly for them to be routinely sought after. In mastectomy specimens a block of nipple should always be examined. The number of lymph nodes recorded in the axilla reflects the time spent on its dissection – there is no doubt that the longer one spends over this task the more nodes one finds (Cuthbert Dukes illustrated this 50 years ago in his method of clearing specimens of rectal carcinoma).

Marrow

Haematological specimens are best shared – marrow imprints or smears can be stained with Leishman's stain then fragments processed to paraffin and into plastic. Diagnosis of haemophagocytosis can be missed if imprints are omitted. Sections of marrow are examined as H & E, MSB, Perls' Scarba Red, and Unna Pappenheim stained preparations.

Lymphoma

Current interest in lymphoma has produced great activity in dealing with nodes and spleen. It seems that new classifications of these cells and their disorders keep appearing in the literature and none is entirely satisfactory. Most lymphoma experts would expect to see ordinary paraffin, plastic embedded and electronmicroscopic preparations as well as immunological ones before reaching a diagnosis.

Lymph nodes

Lymph nodes provide pathologists with many problems as well as satisfying opportunities to impress ones colleagues! – crystals in cystinosis, curious lipogranulomatous reactions to lymphangiographic media, bizarre reactions to drugs (especially the anticonvulsant ones), unexpected infection such as syphilis or cat scratch fever. Special stains such as those for demonstrating reticulin are believed by some to be essential for the proper assessment of a lymph node: they may not shorten the time it takes to arrive at a correct diagnosis and, as with all special staining procedures, results are never as clearcut as one would like. PAS staining is useful in that it covers a whole range of diagnostic changes – mucin-forming carcinoma, glycogen-rich tumours, Waldenstrom's macroglobulinaemia, fungal and amoebic infections and basement membranes.

Bone

It is necessary to decide beforehand whether bone biopsy is to provide decalcified or undecalcified sections – the latter being essential for confident diagnosis of osteomalacia where osteoid seams will be widened and easily assessed on a silver-stained undecalcified section.

Decalcification procedures range from the ultra rapid (RDA) within minutes, to Nitric Acid within hours and EDTA which may take weeks to decalcify thick cortical bone. Thick spicules of bone can be cut on the cryostat so that it is reasonable for an orthopaedic surgeon to ask for an opinion on whether or not he has achieved clearance of a tumour, say in marrow cavity of a long bone.

Examination of bone sections by polarising microscopy is useful in evaluating whether bony trabeculae still retain their lamellar pattern or are replaced by fibrous woven bone. Thus it is of value in diagnosing Paget's disease of bone and fibrous dysplasia. Special stains which we find useful in emphasising the cement lines in bone include PAS Harris' haematoxylin, and MSB gives interesting colour changes which in some way relate to altered bone growth. Yellow-looking bone is worth examination under ultraviolet light – if tetracycline is responsible, the bone will show brilliant fluorescence.

Synovium

Examination of biopsies (needle) of synovium and synovial fluid is becoming more and more requested. Polarising microscopy of a wet preparation (include any clot) allows instant recognition of uric acid/urate crystals in gout (negatively birefringent needles) and pyrophosphatic crystals in pseudogout (positively birefringent rhomboids). Ragocytes (raisin cell) are granular cells found in joint fluid in rheumatoid synovitis.

Muscle

Muscle is the tissue which suffers more than any other when it comes to biopsy. We now believe that using a muscle clamp is the best way to obtain good results, certainly the clamp enables one to take blocks in the right planes and most of the artefacts produced by other methods are avoided. We have not found needle biopsies to be consistently satisfactory. It is essential if one is to carry out histochemical and electronmicroscopic examination as well as light microscopy, that prior notification of the intended biopsy be given so that the person dealing with the specimen is available to cut it (using a half of a safety razor blade) to obtain transverse and longitudinal blocks; some are then placed on cork discs and quenched in isopentane in liquid nitrogen in readiness for cryostat sections, others are processed for electronmicroscopy.

Liver

In generalised liver disorders needle biopsy is now a very common procedure – almost routine – and produces an adequate sample. The quality of histology is improved if the cores are hand processed and special staining for glycogen, reticulin, collagen, haemosiderin and hepatitis virus (orcein) are routine. There are large atlases wholly devoted to this topic.

Gallstones

It is doubtful whether routine quantitative analysis of all gallstones can be justified. Colour, shape and consistency give a good guide as to the composition. Convention lists three forms of stone, 'pure', 'mixed' and 'combined'. 'Pure' stones may be *sterol* (ovoid, solitary and with beautiful crystal formation on the surface which is either transparent white or faintly yellowish as a result of a minimum of bile staining); *pigment* (variable shape, from delicate black twigs of calcium bilirubinate to thick branches or multiple granules sometimes fusing to form bramble-like masses. Calcium carbonate stones are white and hard mulberry-like masses or soft toothpaste-like sludge. The 'mixed' stones have these three constituents intimately intermingled, with one or other predominating and this determines the colour which may range from silvery pearl to black. They show lamination and radial striation and when multiple become facetted with smoothed off angles, or when very numerous, polished and rounded. 'Combined' stones have a core which may be either pure or mixed and a shell of differing composition.

In practice there are several aspects of gallstones worth remembering – cholesterol stones can be made to dissolve while the other types cannot; if one finds a facetted stone in the common bile duct one should look for more; very large gallstones may ulcerate through the gallbladder wall into the small bowel; mucosal metaplasia may occur in the stone-containing gallbladder and carcinoma may supervene; operating to remove gallstones from patients in the over 60 age group is risky with high morbidity and significant mortality.

Gastrointestinal tract

The endoscopic biopsy is the biggest growth industry in pathology laboratories!

Oesophageal mucosa in health shows few intrusive cells and the capillaries and papillae lie low in the epithelium. In chronic oesophagitis the reverse is found. The small fibrescope gastric biopsies pose problems in that the pathologist may be asked to give histological opinion on material which is often traumatised and fit only for a cytological assessment. A similar situation may occur with brain biopsy where a smear may be more informative than a section. Jejunal biopsies (Crosby capsule) can be beautiful when viewed with dissecting microscope or scanning EM. Just how useful an exercise this is in routine practice is uncertain. So many diseases can lead to alteration of mucosal villi that dissecting microscopic observation of villi is unlikely to be diagnostic. Proper quantitation and cell kinetics may prove more useful in the future. Imprints are very informative when stained with Giemsa's stain. Disaccharidase deficiency requires chemical analysis of a fresh biopsy. In cases of suspected Whipple's disease electron-microscopy allows confirmation of the diagnosis through demonstration of the pathognomonic bacillary bodies. Electronmicroscopy is also invaluable in the more precise classification of the APUD series of cells and neoplasms derived from them, size, shape, and number of intracytoplasmic granules being useful parameters. Lead haema-toxylin (Solcia) is useful in paraffin sections for picking out APUD cells, as are modified phloxine methods.

Carcinoid tumours may have a yellow colour which intensifies on fixation in formalin. Numerous staining methods are available for demonstrating argentaffinity (Singh is speedy and gives a clean preparation) and argyrophilia (Holmes). Paneth cells are usually obvious in a well-stained H&E section but can be displayed more vividly using phloxine-tartrazine.

Cytological examination of faeces has become less important now that the fibrescope has brought the whole of the large bowel within view: three common changes seen in biopsies of colonic mucosa are melanosis, aggregation of muciphages, and spirochaetosis. None of these appears to have great clinical importance. Rectal biopsy is a useful convenient method of obtaining tissue for the diagnosis of amyloid disease.

In Hirschsprung's disease cryostat section of a biopsy including mucosa and submucosa can be stained by conventional methods, but demon-stration of ganglion cells is easier in Unna Pappen-heim stained sections or in preparations to show cholinesterase. Neither of these obscures the large abnormal nerve trunks which occur in the disease.

Kidneys

Renal biopsy, like liver biopsy has become a very common investigation. There is no single procedure or method of fixation to cover all the techniques now considered essential, including light micro-scopy (paraffin and plastic) electronmicroscopy, and immunofluorescence. We encourage the clinician to arrange the biopsy so that the scientific officer is available to deal with these immediately, and the remainder of the biopsy is paraffin proces-sed – in addition to H&E sections, we routinely examine thin sections using PACAMS for basement membrane and MSB for fibrin. Techniques for producing satisfactory urinary cytology have improved greatly and it is now possible to give reliable judgements on screening of urine for neoplastic cells in dye workers, etc. The older fashioned examination of urinary deposit is still an important one, for finding casts should certainly make a surgeon think twice before embarking on a surgical course, and finding diagnostic crystals such as cystine can be important.

'Urinary calculi'

Urinary calculi are classified according to com-position, the commonest constituents being calcium oxalate (either monohydrate or dihydrate) calcium phosphate (as carbonate apatite or hydroxyapatite) uric acid and urate, and cystine.

Calcium oxalate stones provide a bewildering variety of colours, shapes and sizes. The dihydrate forms are honey-coloured and spiky as a result of projecting crystals on the surface. The other oxalate stones are often brown to black, laminated or coralline. The smallest ones (less than 1 mm may look like little pearls or hempseed (though with little spines); slightly larger ones may resemble pebbles; some malingering patients may present beach pebbles which they claim to have passed in the urine but their silicate contents gives the game away. Fur from electric kettle is also sometimes passed off as a urinary stone – it is largely carbonate. Other shapes include beetle, cornet, oak apple, jackstone, primula head, and mulberry. Calcium oxalate stones showing lamination are associated with urinary tract infection.

Calcium phosphate stones are pale white or creamy and usually laminated. If solitary, they are ovoid, when multiple they are facetted and they may form a perfect cast of a calyx, pelvis or cavity of the urinary bladder. Infective phosphate often coats foreign bodies and catheters. Randall's plaque refers to the accumulation of calcium salts towards the apex of a pyramid where they may provide a nidus for stone formation.

Uric acid and urate stones are not common: they tend to be varying shades of brown and may be small and rounded especially in the calyces, or large and facetted in the urinary bladder. Solitary huge vesical stones often show attractive lamination resembling an agate. Urate stones are associated with hyperuricaemia so that they complicate gout, polycythaemia, leukemia and other myeloprolifer-ative disorders.

Cystine stones are rare; one form consists of aggregates of hexagonal crystals producing an ovoid large (2 cm to 3 cm) golden stone; another is as facetted whitish tetrahedrons with a soapy feel and tendency to go green with age. They occur in patients who excrete excess cystine, lysine and arginine in the urine. Alkalinisation of the urine is said to be of prophylactic value.

Any patient with urinary stone must have blood analysed for calcium, phosphate, uric acid plasma protein and electrolytes; it is also wise to have an xray of hands and skull.

Conditions associated with calcium-containing stones include – hypercalcaemia and hypercalcuria as in hyperparathyroidism Vitamin-D intoxication, hyperthyroidism, immobilisation, milk-alkali syndrome, sarcoidosis, Paget's disease of bone, myelomatosis and carcinomatosis; hyperoxaluria as in Crohn's disease; obstruction and stasis in urinary tract; infection with urea splitting organisms; foreign bodies; analgesic nephropathy with sloughed papilla acting as a nidus; and geographic factors such as climate, diet, parasites, water, drugs, and social customs.

Analysis of semen

Seminal analysis is now requested routinely as a follow-up check on vasectomy; such requests now outnumber those for investigations of infertility. Normally seminal fluid (2 to 5 ml) contains over 40 million spermatozoa per ml, with motile forms outnumbering nonmotile and in a stained smear there should be fewer than 40 per cent abnormal forms. Azoospermia refers to absence of spermatozoa which is most commonly caused by disordered spermatogenesis either aplasia, maturation arrest, conducting system obstruction, or by post-inflammatory atrophy. Oligospermia refers to a reduction in number below the normal: rarely if the sufferer has a varicocoele its cure may improve the sperm count.

Testes

Testicular biopsy is done in infertile patients who have been shown to have significant reduction in spermatozoa and in a variety of cases with suspected chromosomal abnormalities. Examination of stained scrapings of buccal epithelium is useful in demonstrating the sex chromatin particle on the nuclear membrane of females, and in stained blood films the drumstick body can be seen in neutrophil polymorphonuclear leucocytes. Biopsy is not recommended for malignant tumours of the testis – these are best dealt with by orchidectomy. Clinically it is very important to examine the testis in all patients in whom a diagnosis of retroperitoneal tumour is made, because seminoma can produce large metastases in the para-aortic nodes; the prognosis with treatment is far better than for most primary retroperitoneal malignant neoplasms.

Endometrium

Endometrium, obtained by curettage or suction is normally transferred straight into fixative for paraffin processing. The more information given to the pathologist the more helpful is his report likely to be. Details of the menstrual cycle and whether the patient is on contraceptive pill should always be given. In the patient under investigation for infertility it is still worthwhile sending part of the fresh tissue for bacteriological examination for mycobacteria and neisseria – if assessment of ovulation is to be reliable the specimen should be taken in the second half of the cycle. In suspected ectopic pregnancy the endometrium is not a reliable guide to diagnosis, though finding Arias-Stella nuclear changes is suggestive. In cases of suspected uterine abortion demonstration of foetal or placental tissue is essential for definite diagnosis. Giant cells in the placental bed often cause problems – they may derive from muscle, decidua, placenta or histiocytes.

Cervix

Cone biopsies of cervix uteri generate a great deal of work for pathologists. It is very important that a reasonable compromise be reached so that other routine requirements do not suffer. Dividing the opened out cone into 3 mm to 4 mm thick blocks and taking sections at three levels suffices for most cases. If cytologically the diagnosis of carcinoma has been made and these sections fail to show the expected lesion, reversing the blocks and taking further sections is justified.

Fibroid

Fibroids of the uterus, if large, present problems as to how many blocks should be examined – in this situation, as in large prostate glands, it is quite exceptional for patients, in whom say an average of up to six blocks has been taken, to return with malignancy attributable to the allegedly benign lesion.

Endometrial carcinoma

In uterine carcinoma, as in other visceral malignancies depth of invasion and node involvements appear to correlate well with survival though the remarkable difference in prognosis between squamous carcinoma of cervix and adenocarcinoma of endometrium should alert one to the shortcomings of grading and staging.

Abortion

In any abortus a proportion of the chorionic villi will show degenerative changes. Commonly there may be swollen hydropic villi without central liquefaction or trophoblastic overgrowth which are the hallmarks of hydatidiform mole. In non-criminal abortion it is perfectly normal to find areas of decidual necrosis, haemorrhage and neutrophil polymorphonuclear leucocytic infiltration. The diagnosis of post-partum infection is best achieved by culture as is that of gonococcal salpingo-oophoritis.

Fallopian tubes

Fallopian tube segments removed at sterilisation are usually straightforward but those taken shortly after delivery commonly show decidual change either on the serosa or in the mucosa. Threadworms do seem to get caught up in the fronds and cause granulomatous salpingitis. Ectopic pregnancy is usually obvious but at times it may require many sections to demonstrate chorionic villi or trophoblastic cells in the blood clot.

Ovary

Ovarian endometriosis may also require a long search for stroma plus the epithelium to substantiate the diagnosis which is usually suggested by the adhesions and haemosiderin-containing phagocytes or chocolate cysts. The ovary is another site which seems to attract threadworms. Ovarian neoplasms often prove difficult to diagnose or give a reliable prognostication particularly papillary tumours in young patients. The question of whether metastatic or primary often arises and generally if the lesions are predominantly cystic, then they are likely to be primary. No reliable way of distinguishing primary and secondary carcinoid tumour of the ovary exists at the moment. Thecoma is usually instantly recognisable by its yellow colour in a fibromatous-looking mass, but a cryostat section examined with the polarising microscope will confirm the presence of the birefringent lipid in the cells. Granulosa cell tumour tends to recur and remain within the abdomen and it, with thecoma appears to provoke endometrial hyperplasia and neoplasia in a proportion of patients. Dermoid cysts may be bilateral and are usually benign. The Stein-Leventhal syndrome ovary shows multiple cortical cysts of follicular type. Other cysts include luteal, serosal and developmental.

Pituitary gland

Biopsy diagnosis of chromophobe adenoma is usually easy but we have seen an example looking very like a plasmacytoma. We use the OFG method to demonstrate eosinophil cells in the adenomas. It is doubtful whether pituitary neoplasms ever metastasize other than locally.

Adrenal glands

When adrenalectomy was done as part of an endocrine ablation for breast cancer, it was common to find metastatic carcinoma in the specimens. Adrenal tumours include cortical adenoma and phaeochromocytoma of the medulla. Although these have quite different origins and functions they may be very difficult to distinguish even with special fixation and special stains. Neuroblastoma is usually readily recognised. Tuberculosis still has to be reckoned with and we have seen one case of histoplasmosis die with adrenal failure caused by granulomatous destruction.

Carotid body

Carotid body tumour and chemodectoma in the region of the middle ear (glomus tumour) have a distinctive histology which makes for easy recognition if the possibility is considered. The problem arises in the ear where the lesion is not recognised clinically (not all cases produce severe bleeding) and no biopsy is taken. Electron microscopy now makes it possible to identify these neoplasms with certainty.

Thyroid gland

More problems probably arise from cryostat sections of thyroid neoplasm than from any other site, with the possible exception of tumours at the lower end of the common bile duct. This is partly because one is only seeing part of the lesion the behaviour of which does not always relate well with the cytological features and the prognostic indicators of capsular penetration, invasion of blood vessels and lymphatics are unlikely to be present in small biopsies and certainly not in needle cores. A further problem arises with hyperplastic thyroid glands which can look very highly cellular, mitotically active and show considerable nuclear pleomorphism. Similarly glands involved with thyroiditis may show remarkable epithelial abnormalities and cellular round cell infiltration.

Papillary neoplasms too provide much speculation and the concept of lateral aberrant thyroid still provokes much argument. The request for an urgent diagnosis on a thyroid neoplasm should always be met with optimistic reserve; it is better for the patient with borderline lesions, whether epithelial or lymphoid, to await good paraffin sections and, if necessary, second opinion. This does not diminish in any way the help that can be given to the surgeons in confirming for him that a benign lesion is benign and vice versa. Calcispherite formation seems to occur with greater frequency in carcinoma than in adenoma but this is rarely of assistance in arriving at a diagnosis in an individual case.

Parathyroid glands

Parathyroidectomy produces usually adenomas which are fairly simple to identify; the main difficulty arises in enlarged glands in which one is faced with nodules of varied structure and asked to decide whether they are neoplastic or not; experience proves that no reliable method is available at the moment. Diffuse hyperplasia with clear cell pattern is sufficiently distinctive for immediate recognition; not so the rare parathyroid carcinoma where, like in thyroid, one needs to demonstrate invasion and metastases before one can really be sure. The case of much mitotic activity in hyperplastic parathyroid glands removed at midnight raises a question (to which we have found no answer) – Is this a physiological phenomenon?

Thymus

Thymectomy is fortunately rare; there are no special techniques required in arriving at a diagnosis of neoplasm which occurs in 15 per cent of cases of myasthenia gravis. Remember that only one-third of thymomas are associated with myasthenia and that they may be locally aggressive and pleural involvement is common. Thymic hyperplasia with active medullary germinal centres is seen in about 75 per cent of the younger cases of myasthenia gravis and only one-third of these show autoantibody compared with 95 per cent of patients with thymoma.

Pancreas

Satisfactory biopsies of pancreas are difficult to obtain technically and this is reflected in the quality of specimens received in the laboratory. With the interest in APUD cells and their neoplasms it is important to have electron microscopy done if an endocrine lesion is suspected. Of course, one may not have an isolated tumour but several tumours or a diffuse cell hyperplasia and the assessment of the latter calls for experience and good quantitative control – not a very easy thing to achieve. Needle aspirates of malignant lesions are fraught with pitfalls for the unwary – one may aspirate material like pus and yet there may still be a carcinoma in the organ.

Central nervous system

Biopsies from the central nervous system require particular attention if the opportunity to diagnose the less common degenerations and disease processes is not to be missed. We believe that for most neurological specimens fixation of part for electron microscopy, part for paraffin section and part for cryostat section or smear cytology covers most of the current requirements. Viral infections such as herpes are certainly diagnosable by culture, by immunological and electron microscopic methods. The range of appearances in primary brain tumours especially in children makes it almost impossible for the ordinary routine pathologist to make consistently correct diagnosis; haemangioblastoma of the cerebellum can be very easily confused with metastatic hypernephroma; meningioma can look very like neurilemmoma or chemodectoma – alkaline phosphatase staining may help; cytology of cerebrospinal fluid may be very informative in infections, infarctions and neoplasms including those long surviving leukaemic patients.

Eyes

The eye is another organ with a bewildering range of pathological problems. Processing can be done either in paraffin or low-viscosity nitrocellulose and still allow tissue to be taken for electron microscopy. As in neuropathology there is quite understandably a reluctance on the part of the general surgical pathologist to get caught up in trabecular meshworks and filtration angles. However, it is a fascinating area and one where correlation between what is seen via the ophthalmoscope and the microscope can be particularly rewarding.

Ears

The ears provide mainly polyps and tissue from middle ear; the former are usually straightforward though on two occasions we have reported polyps consisting of herniated cerebrum and once a polyp which turned out to be a chemodectomatous prolongation. The tissues from the middle ear are usually stapes (or parts of stapes) requiring histological confirmation of otosclerosis to show Pagetoid changes, or plaques of acellular collagenous tissue which characterise tympanosclerosis. These requests can be dealt with by routine decalcified paraffin processing. Metastatic carcinoma does occur in middle ear – in our experience from primary carcinoma of breast and bronchus and from malignant melanoma.

Fungus

While fungus is literally in the territory of the microbiologist, it is often the histopathologist who first raises the possibility from appearances in routine paraffin sections. Identification of the type of fungus requires culture or other bacteriological techniques. The pathologist has many special stains which render the organisms more conspicuous and may well suggest a particular group (aspergillus in lung, actinomyces in neck, histoplasma in the tongue, or mucor in the orbit). These stains are also helpful in picking up sparse fungal elements in granulomas, especially the Grocott Methenamine Silver.

Index

Index

The numbers in **bold** indicate figure numbers; the figures in medium-face type indicate page numbers.

228